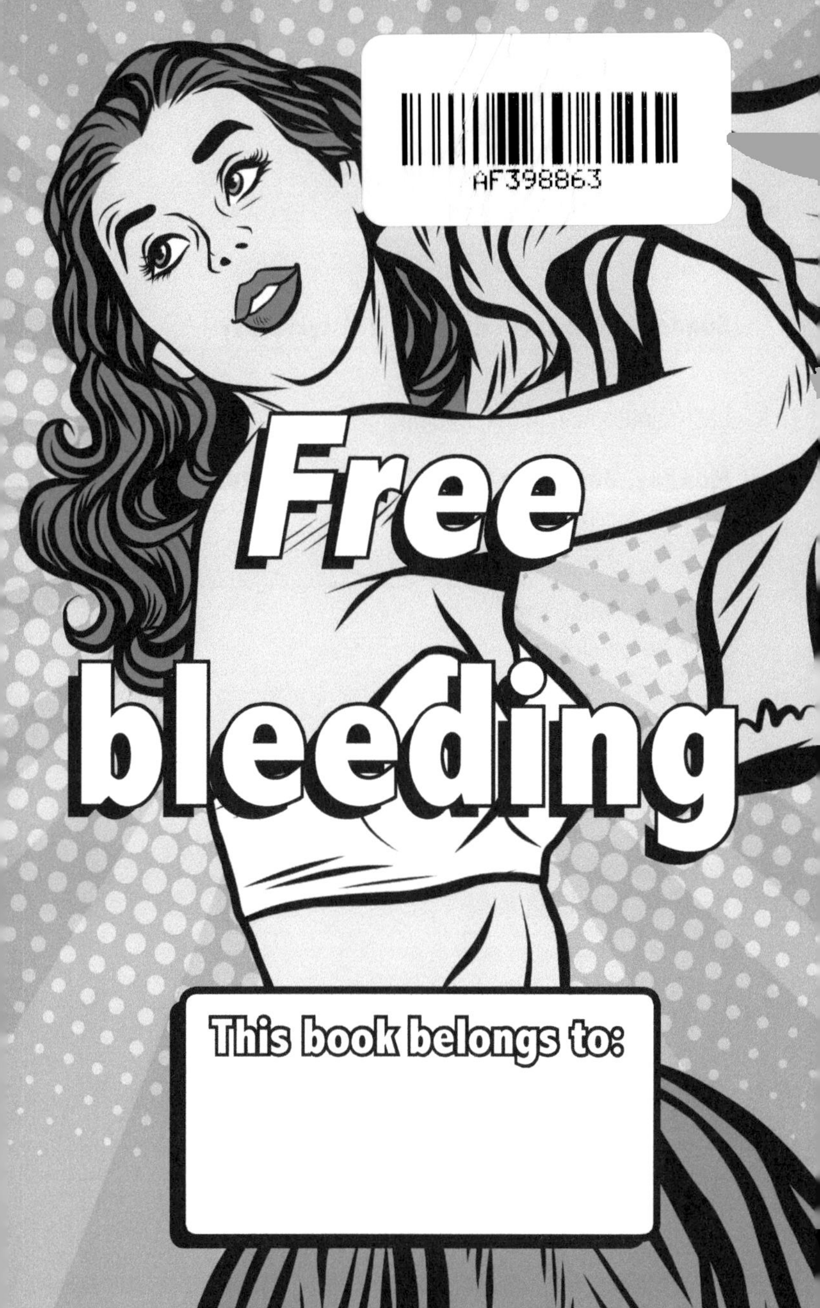
AF398863
Free bleeding
This book belongs to:

Contents

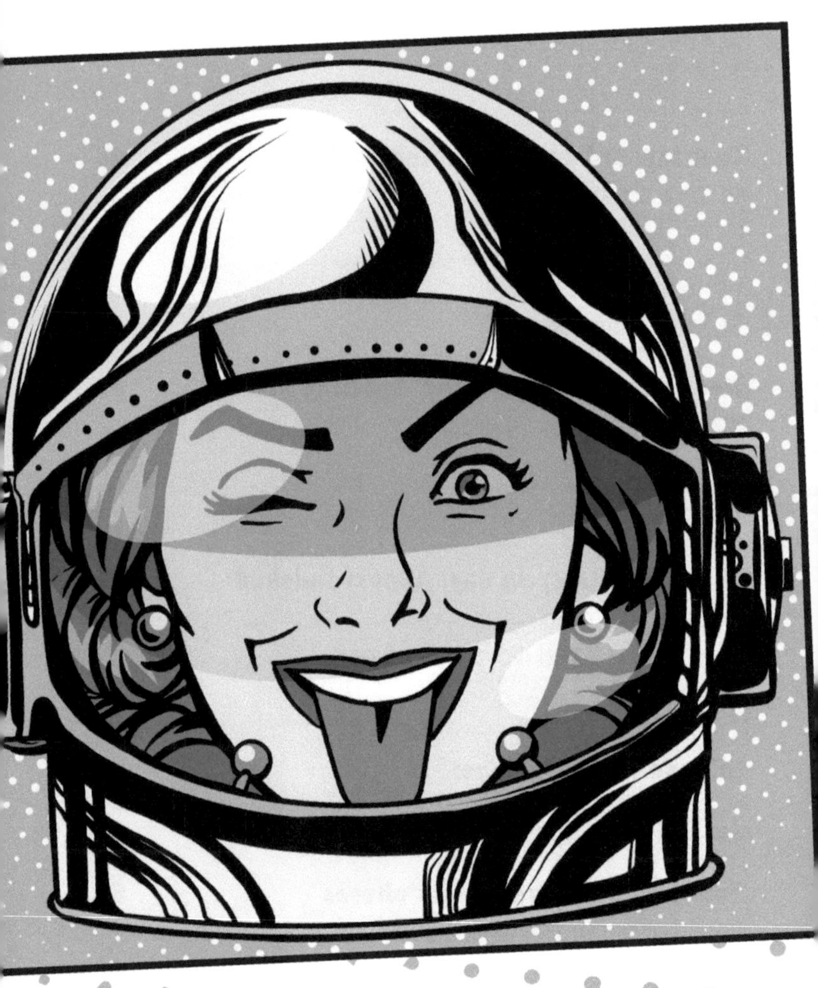

This is Lea.

Lea is 32 years old, married with two daughters whom she gave birth to at home. One girl is at primary school, the other still crawls into Mummy's bed at night.

Lea is a freelance advertising expert and works from her home office. This is a practical set-up, as it means she usually always has free access to a toilet. It's an unbeatable advantage for having a stress-free product-free period, which Lea has done for several years.

As Lea doesn't just want to design and write the advertising campaign for the first manned Mars mission, she has also allowed us to follow along with her free bleeding in this COMIC DIARY which she wrote especially for us.

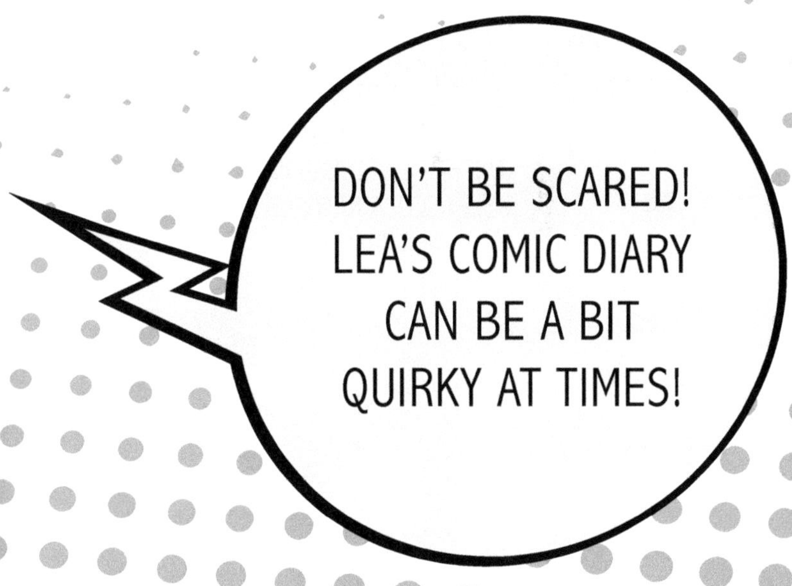

Periods – what are they?

Before we start, let's quickly summarise what it's all about.

When a girl reaches a certain age, she becomes a woman who can become pregnant. The special thing about this is that your uterus bleeds now and then, and this blood flows out of the vagina.

Different hormones ensure that bleeding occurs regularly. This is why it's also called "monthlies" or your "period". It can also be called "menstruation" because the bleeding occurs approximately every 28 days, which is about once a month (from the Latin "mens").

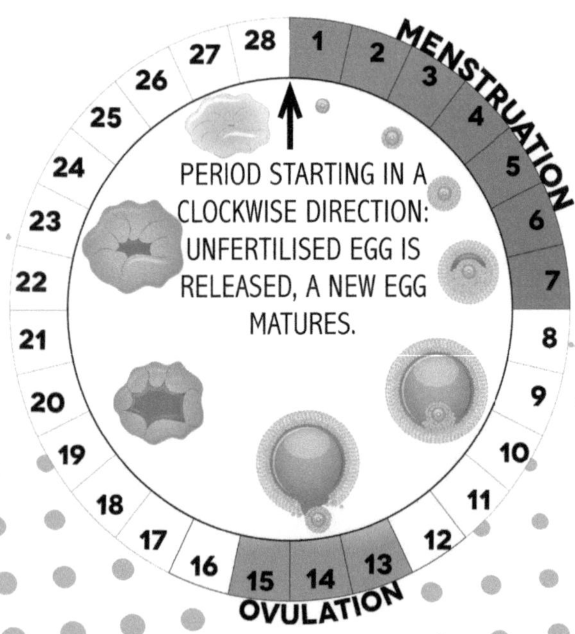

Your body wants to ensure you have the chance to reproduce every month.

The egg, from which a baby could develop, 'jumps' from one of your two ovaries into one of the fallopian tubes found to the left and right of the womb during ovulation ("ovulation" from Latin, ovus = egg). Some women feel their ovulation during this time directly to the left or right below the navel.

You are fertile and can become pregnant, even several days before ovulation occurs. You can detect this fertile period by checking your vaginal discharge which becomes stretchier until it feels like egg white.

If an egg is not fertilised during sex by the man's ejaculate which contains sperm, then it does not need to be anchored to the moist mucus membrane of the womb.

In this case, your body realises you are not pregnant and vigorously pushes out the unfertilised egg from your uterus, together with the old mucus membrane: You bleed and all the old materials are eliminated.

In healthy women, this cycle takes place automatically. Except for when you are pregnant, breastfeeding or taking a pill or other hormones which supress ovulation (so-called "ovulation inhibitors").

What is free bleeding?

Free bleeding is when you have a period without (many) tampons, sanitary towels, menstrual cups, sponges or other hygiene products and instead allow the blood to flow out "freely".

Being able to manage your period easily without feeling stuffed up or having to have sanitary towels in your pants is a big relief - particularly when it comes to annoying period pains. Many women and girls feel considerably more free and self-reliant than before.

Why? It's simple: Allowing your body to bleed freely means,

...   you know what's going on inside your body. This means you are naturally more open and relaxed than when you are only using tampons or sanitary towels.

...   you are no longer completely dependent on commercial period products. This allows you to take the lead and become more self-reliant about your body because you can manage without visiting the chemist.

...   you follow your body's rhythm. This usually allows everything to get into a better swing and you can even accelerate your cycle, thereby shortening the time you bleed for.

...   last but not least, you feel and support the power of your uterus. This muscle is very powerful and can even give birth to your child! Having a period free of products is therefore good training for having an easy birth. And just like when giving birth, the tensing and relaxing of the uterus does not hurt.

It also goes without saying that it is far more environmentally friendly and cheaper to use only a few sheets of toilet paper to protect your clothes instead of using a new disposable sanitary towel or a tampon each time.

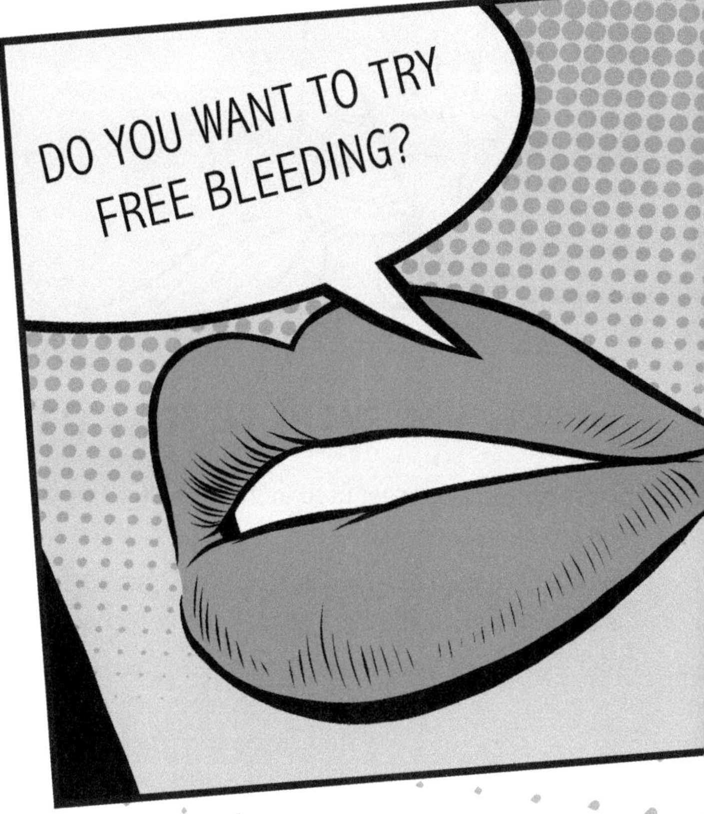

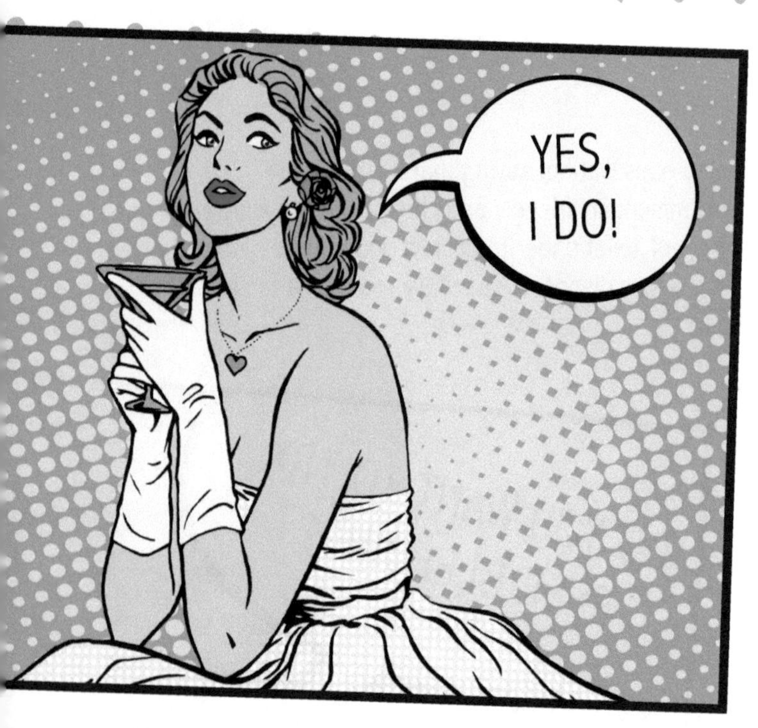

Great, you want to take part!

Most people usually get used to free bleeding after a couple of practice cycles.

So if you're keen on experimenting, rest assured that you will become more and more used to this very practical method over time.

However, even for experienced free bleeding practitioners, there are always key questions on how to put a product-free period into practice, e.g.:

...	How will I know when my period is starting and when it's over?

...	What do I do when I'm on the go?

...	Will I leak in the night?

...	How often will I need to go to the toilet on heavy flow days?

...	Can I swim or use a sauna on product-free period days?

All of these questions can be answered.

Ideally by someone who already has lots of experience with this method. This is why Lea has noted down her flow for one cycle, writing down when she is not using tampons or sanitary towels for absorbance - at home and on the go.

To make sure Lea remembered every little detail, she created the FREE BLEEDING DIARY, which her children found very amusing. Because who writes a report on what they're doing in the toilet?

Writing it down is a good idea. This allows you to keep an eye on your research results and note down your OWN recipe for product-free period success alongside Lea's description.

It is best to see for yourself which days and for which requirements you prefer having a product-free period with a combination of other "classic methods".

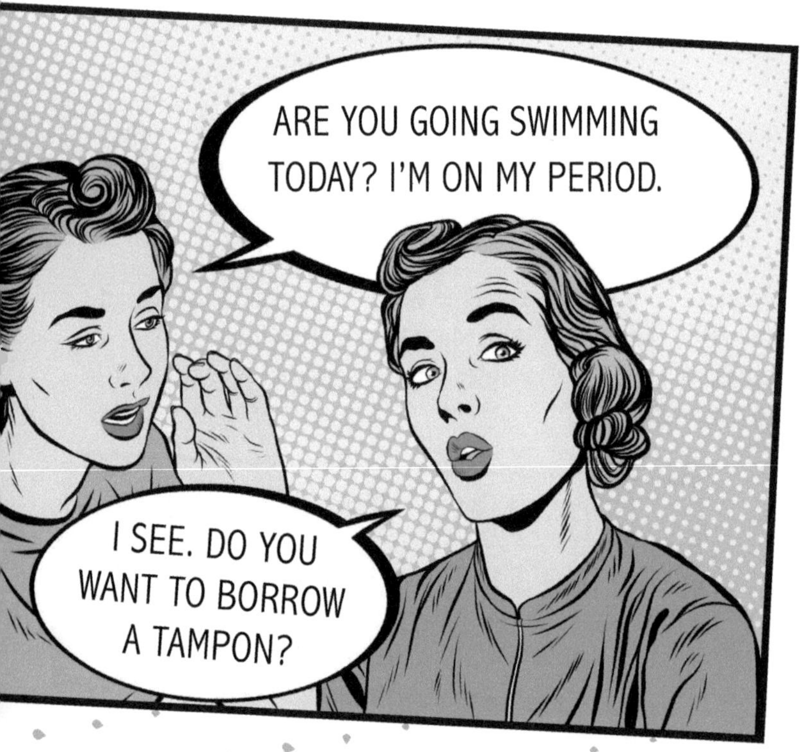

You can forgo your product-free period, e.g. when swimming, in the sauna or on the go for a long time by using traditional products like tampons, sanitary towels etc., and then easily go back to free bleeding.

The good thing about it: Once you have learned about and practiced having a product-free period, you an always 'activate' it again. You can of course also use products sometimes, part-time, or even go an entire cycle on conventional products.

You always retain your knowledge about free bleeding, just as you know you won't suddenly forget how to brush your teeth if you neglect to brush them one morning.

Have fun with Lea's story and menstruating without (many) sanitary towels, tampons, etc.!

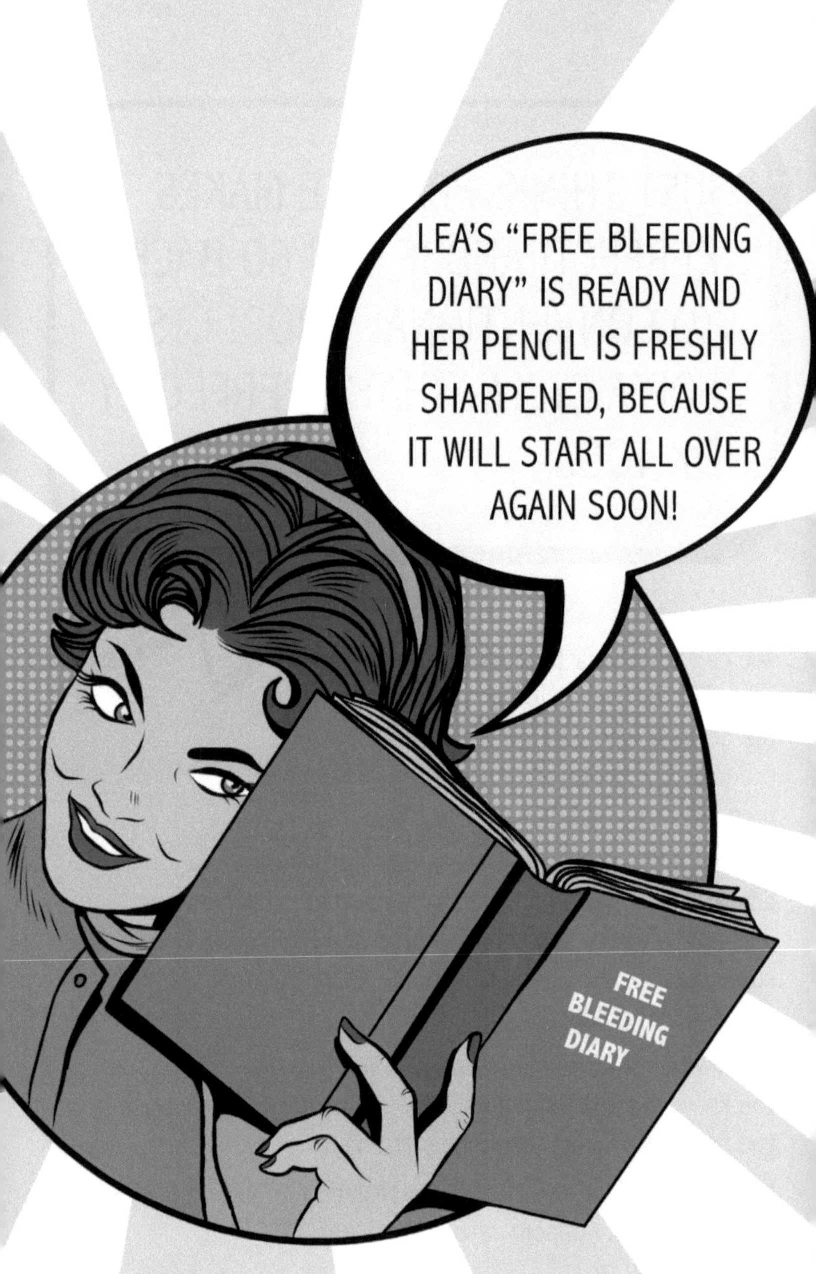

LEA'S "FREE BLEEDING DIARY" IS READY AND HER PENCIL IS FRESHLY SHARPENED, BECAUSE IT WILL START ALL OVER AGAIN SOON!
FREE BLEEDING DIARY

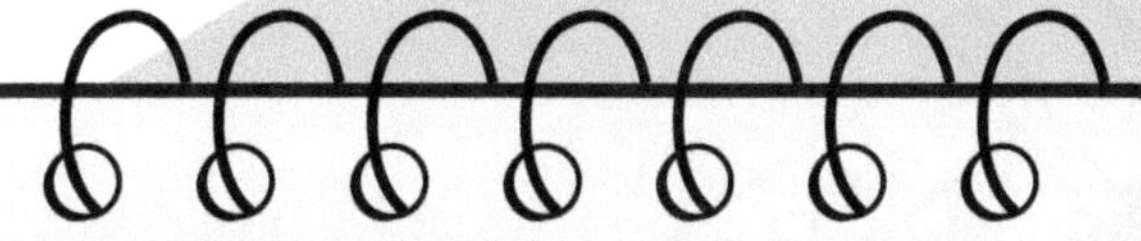

Sunday, 29th cycle day and 1st cycle day

9PM

I go to the toilet and see that there's some blood on the toilet paper.

Although it's already late in the evening, I decide to count today/this evening as my 1st cycle day. Blood is blood, after all.

I suspect my waking temperature* today has already fallen by a few tenths of a degree, which marks the real start of my cycle. However, I haven't measured it as I've been tired from several breastfeeding sessions overnight.

There is still not much coming out.

Nevertheless, I put three sheets of toilet paper into my pants as I don't know how fast it will come on.

*Lea usually measures her waking temperature to maintain full control over her cycle. If you want to find out more about it and want to measure your own cycle, you can get the "My Time of the Month" Cycle Diary.

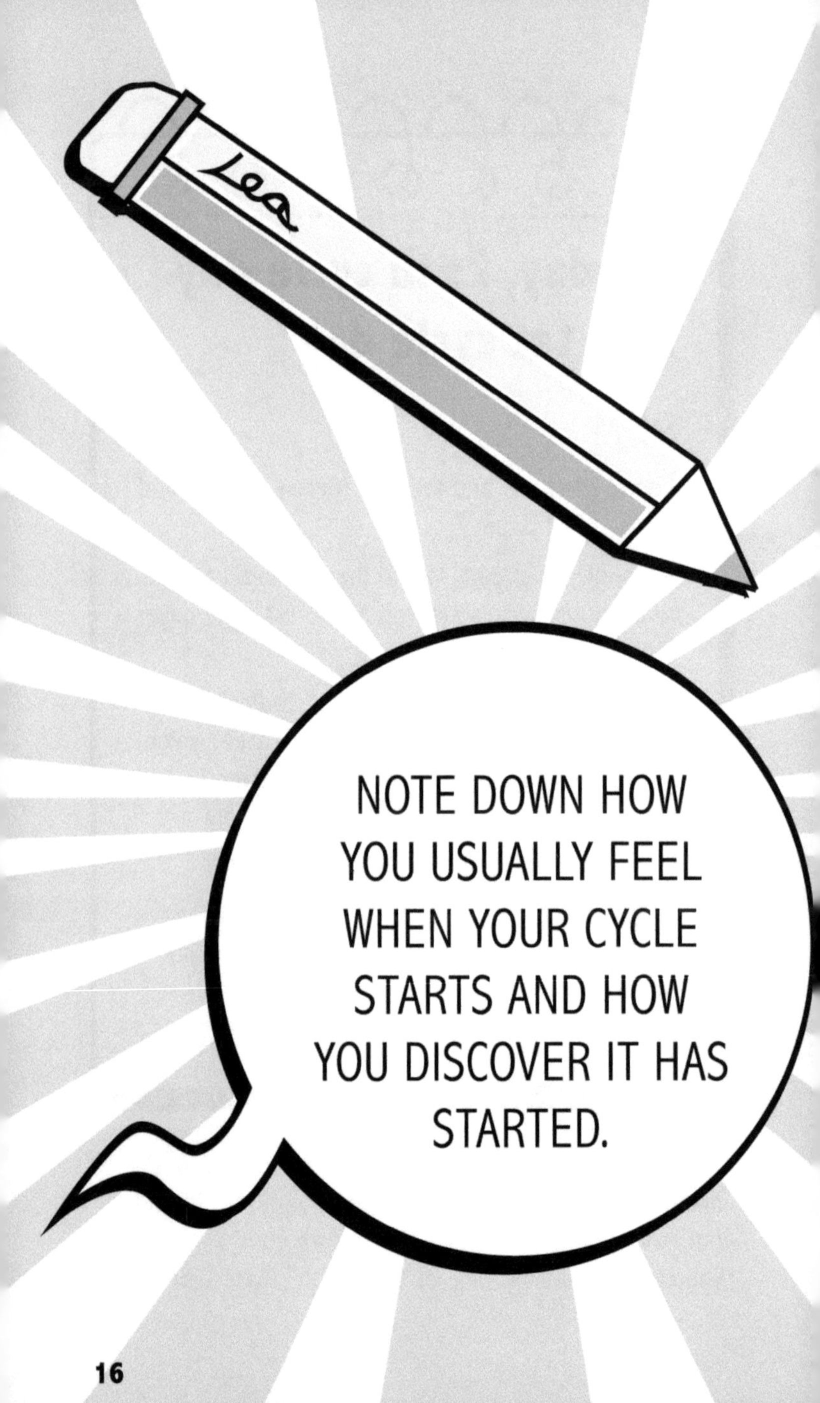

NOTE DOWN HOW
YOU USUALLY FEEL
WHEN YOUR CYCLE
STARTS AND HOW
YOU DISCOVER IT HAS
STARTED.

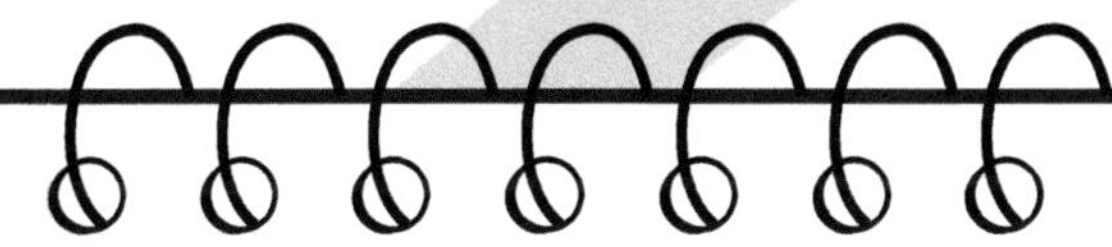

What do you know about the start of your cycle?

☐ Sometimes I get blood on my pants which is really annoying.

☐ I measure my temperature every morning and realise that it is coming before bleeding starts.

☐ I'm a bit bloated and moody before my cycle starts.

☐ On the days before my period I take things easy as I am more sensitive than usual.

☐ ....

....

☐ ....

....

☐ ....

....

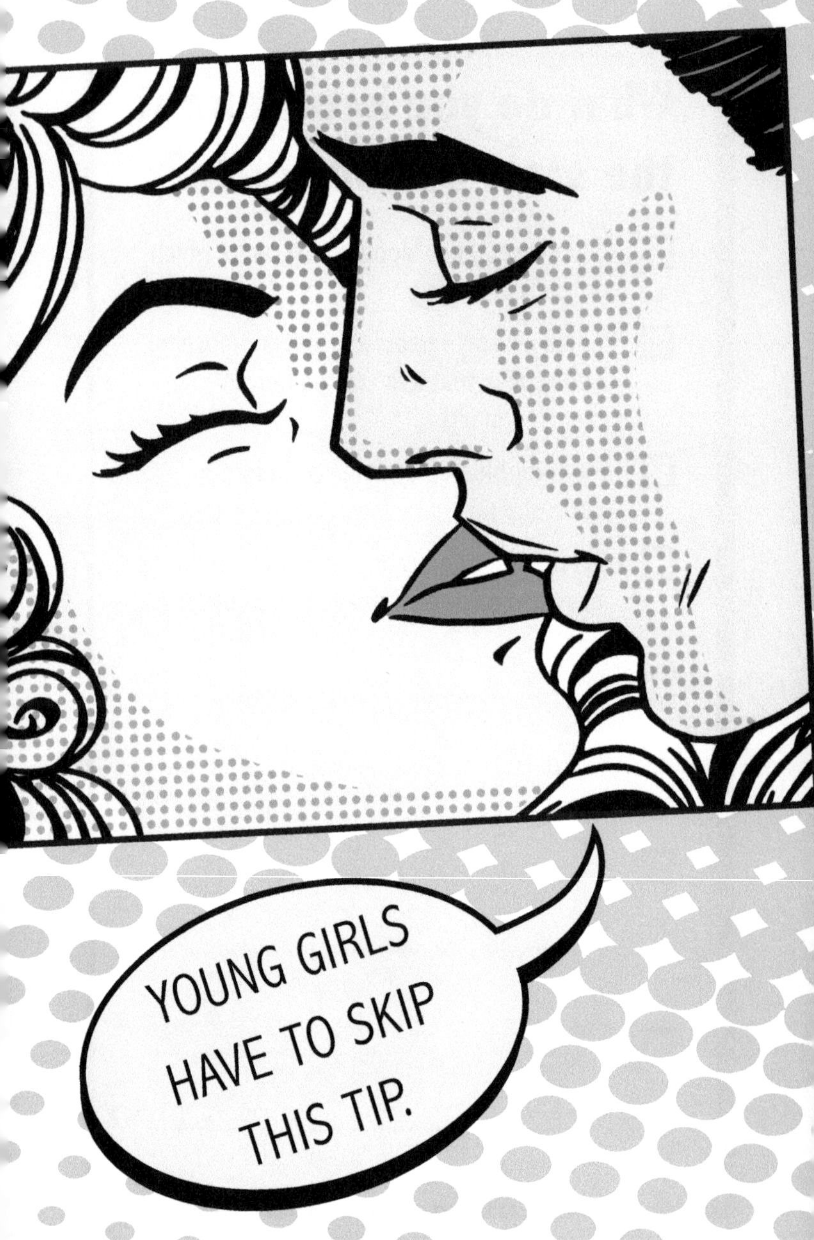

YOUNG GIRLS HAVE TO SKIP THIS TIP.

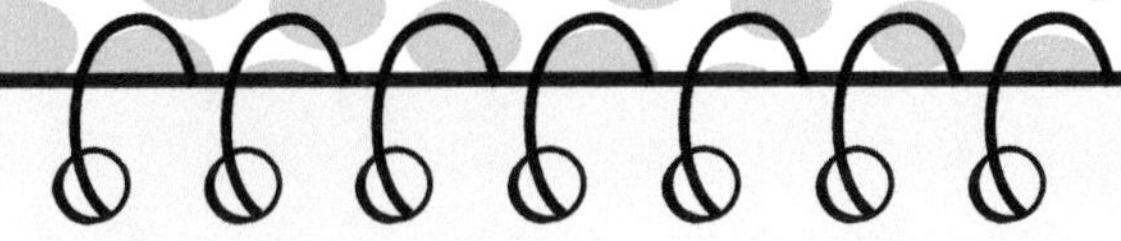

Last minute menstruation help

It's rare, but still: I actually spent a cosy night on the sofa watching television with my husband.

It is half past eleven at night. The film is over and lots of knights died. But they managed to conquer the palace. Well, those who survived did.

Knights ... good idea! They are strong, valiant and always ready to do heroic things. Just like my husband.

Late at night, I get him to also play a knight and be my early menstruation helper.

How? Sex! His sperm contains prostaglandins which facilitate the opening of my cervix.

Similar to childbirth. He was just as heroic in undertaking this difficult task when our second child came into the world ;-)

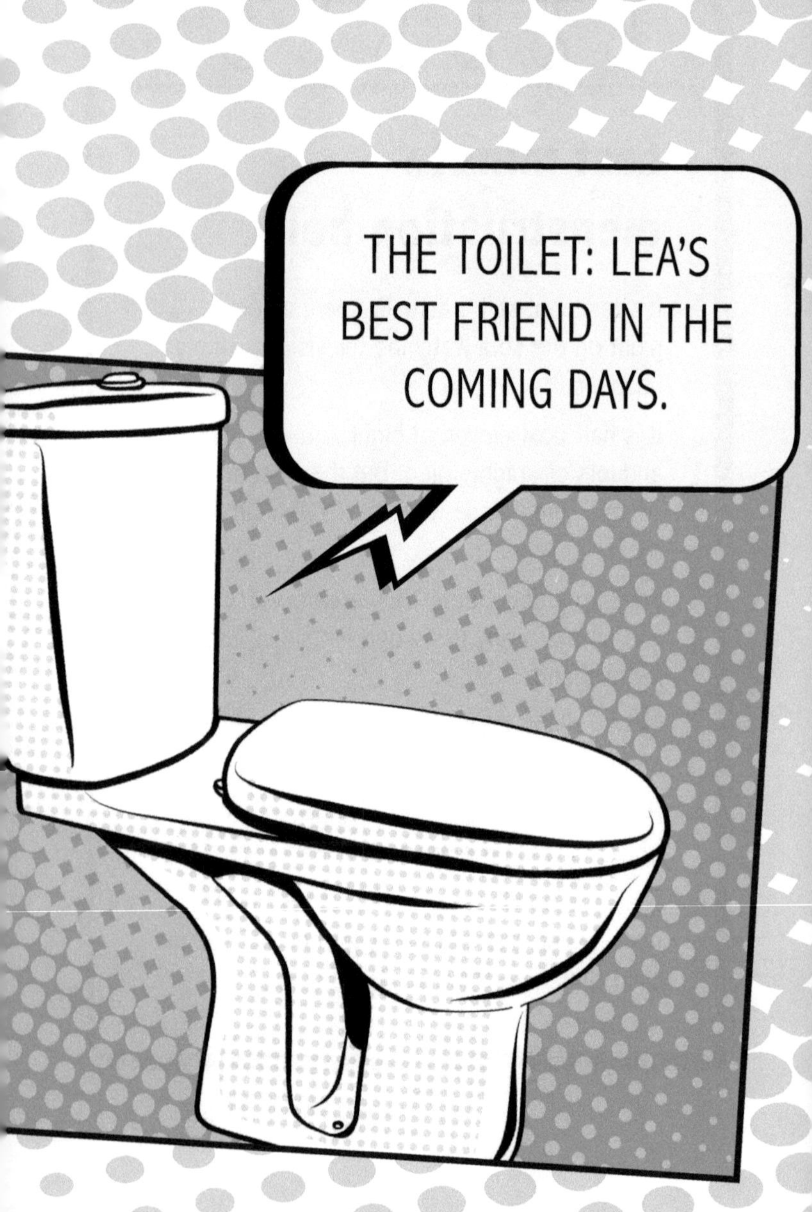

THE TOILET: LEA'S BEST FRIEND IN THE COMING DAYS.

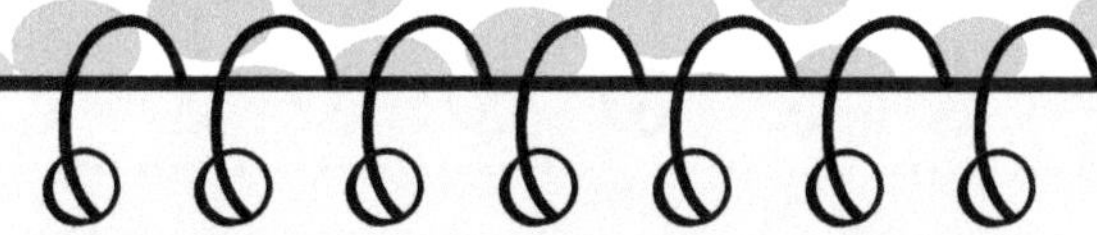

Monday, 2nd cycle day: Night time disturbance

3AM

Our youngest gets into our bed with kit and caboodle. It's a tight squeeze and uncomfortable.

At times like this I wake up and need the loo, just like I do now. Half asleep, I think: Right, my period can start now.

As I don't want to turn on the light, I feel inside myself. It feels damp, even where no wee runs down.

I sit on the loo for a bit longer just to be on the safe side.

After half a minute or so, I squat down, push down a bit and clean myself.

In the semi-darkness I see a few blood stains. I wipe the area again and put some folded sheets of toilet paper into my pants, which I am wearing under my pyjama bottoms.

Monday morning: Hurry up now!

8.40AM

Today is a holiday. How practical on the first real day of my cycle!

I will need to go to the toilet frequently.

When I wake up or am woken up by my child, who wants to use the potty, I also feel the need to go to the toilet. I am looking forward to an impressive yield, because a lot could have accumulated over the last few hours.

Curious, I look at the water stream. As expected, I see a thick strand of menstrual blood. For a few seconds it runs alongside the pale yellow urine, then drips out on its own.

To get rid of the menstrual blood completely, like I want to do right now, I go down into a deep squat after urinating and tilt my pelvis forwards slightly.

I bear down and rest, bear down and rest and some more menstrual fluid comes out.

Then, after about a minute on the toilet, the dripping stops and I wipe myself off. There is of course still some blood on the toilet paper, mixed with urine, but not that much.

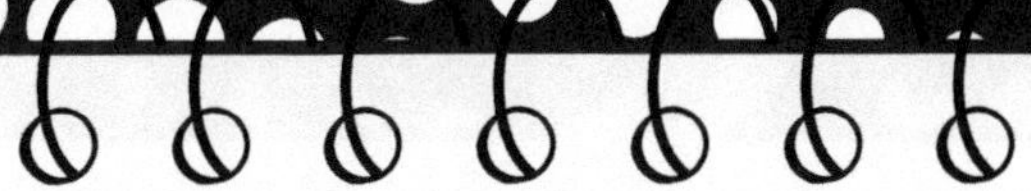

That's enough for the moment; after cleaning up I put a few folded sheets of toilet paper into my knickers.

If I were going to leave the house straight away today, on the first heavy day of my cycle, I would put a thin panty liner into my pants and then the folded toilet paper over it. Because when you're on the go you don't always know where the next clean toilet will be.

TOILET PAPER — TP FOR SHORT — PROTECTS BOTH YOUR PANTS AND YOUR PANTY LINER IF YOU WANT TO USE ONE FOR PEACE OF MIND.

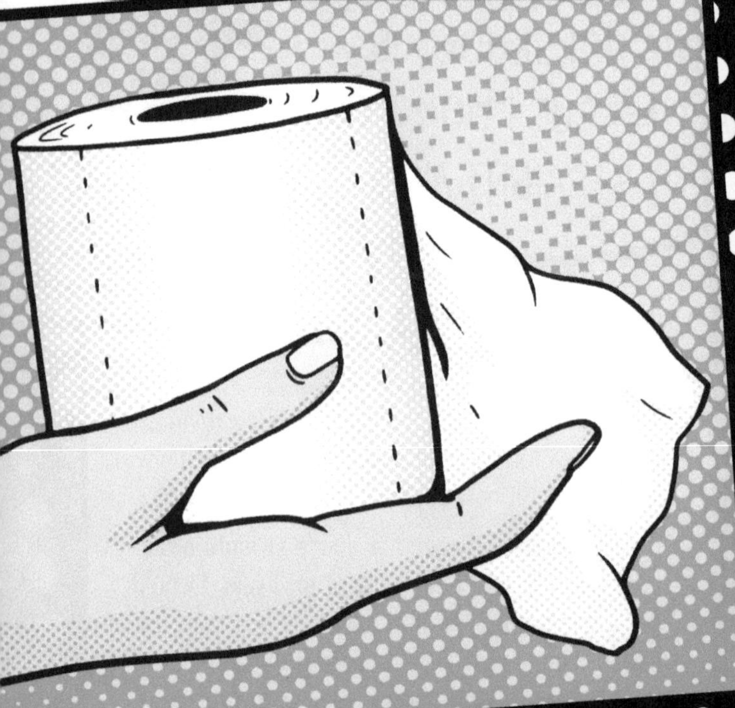

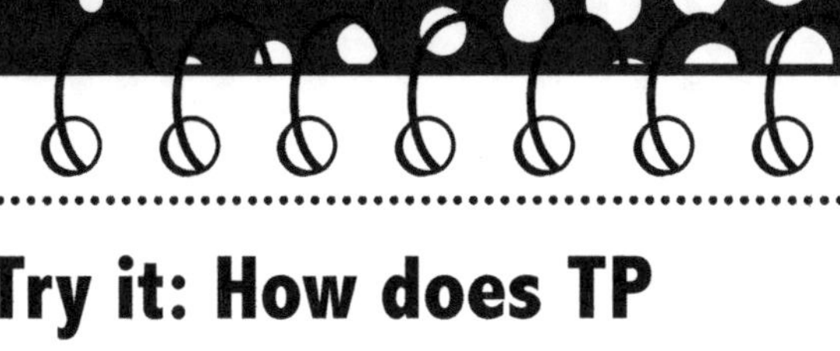

Try it: How does TP work for you?

- ☐   Great, it's a really good idea!
- ☐   I find TP too scratchy. I use softer paper and get some fluffy rolls of TP or several packs of soft tissues.
- ☐   It feels a bit strange, but I might be able to get used to it.
- ☐   ....
....
- ☐   ....
....
- ☐   ....
....

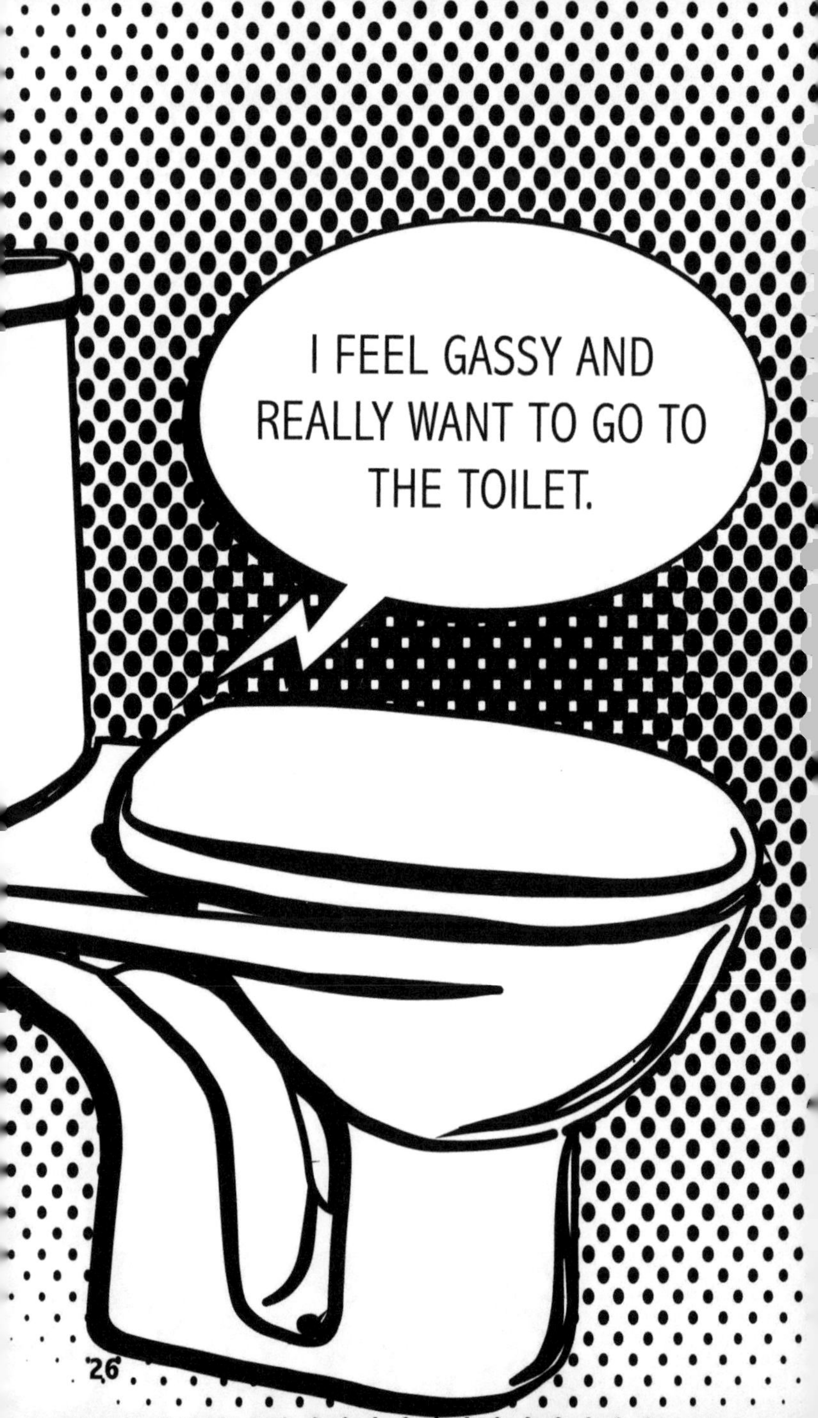

I FEEL GASSY AND
REALLY WANT TO GO TO
THE TOILET.

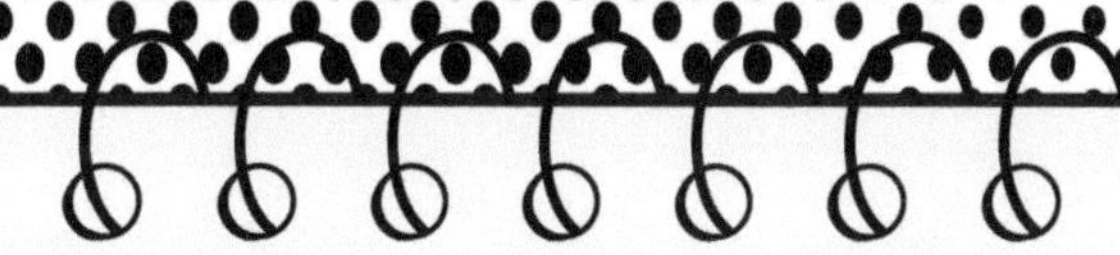

Bloating... what now?

9.20AM

A powerful bowel movement at the beginning of the cycle is coming! I used to be blindsided by this: As a young girl I didn't yet know that the start of your period and having a big bowel movement were connected.

I quickly go to the loo because I know that something liquid needs to come out.

Yikes! A little torrent of blood has landed in my pants and soaked through the toilet paper. Well, it's not so bad. I'll wash out the blood afterwards with COLD WATER.

I sit on the toilet so that my toes are raised and my torso is slightly tilted forwards. This allows my bowels to do their work more easily.

Whilst my business moves down towards the sewerage system beneath me, I feel the pressure in my abdomen subside. It's nice because I don't have any more pain.

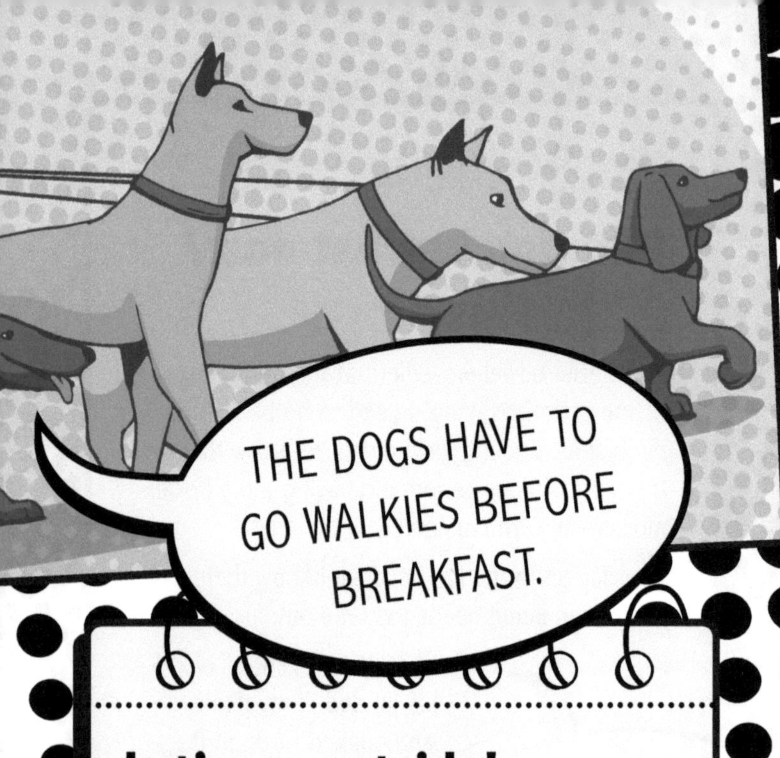

Let's go outside!
9.30AM

How long will I need? No idea. Perhaps my children will dawdle.

After cleaning up, I change my underwear:

I pick out black pants, put in a thin panty liner and lay four sheets of folded toilet paper over it. I also choose to wear BLACK clothes. Better safe than sorry.

I quickly wash my slightly bloodied pants in COLD WATER. This washes off the spot of blood.

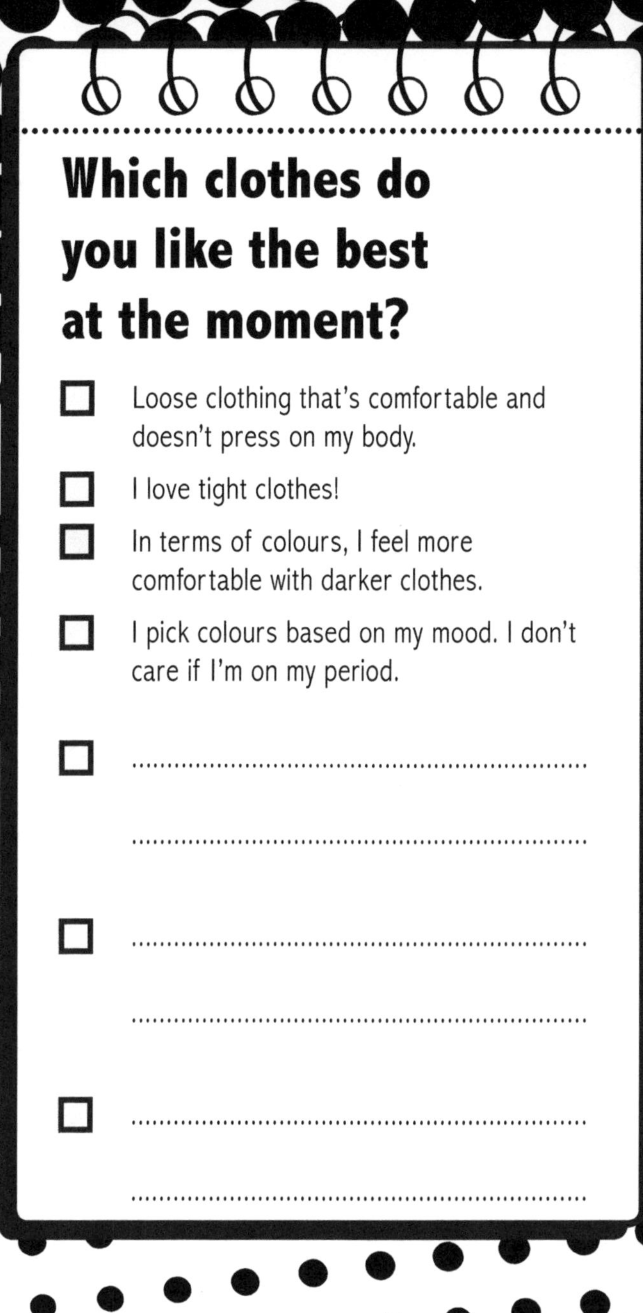

Which clothes do you like the best at the moment?

- ☐ Loose clothing that's comfortable and doesn't press on my body.
- ☐ I love tight clothes!
- ☐ In terms of colours, I feel more comfortable with darker clothes.
- ☐ I pick colours based on my mood. I don't care if I'm on my period.
- ☐ ....
  ....
- ☐ ....
  ....
- ☐ ....
  ....

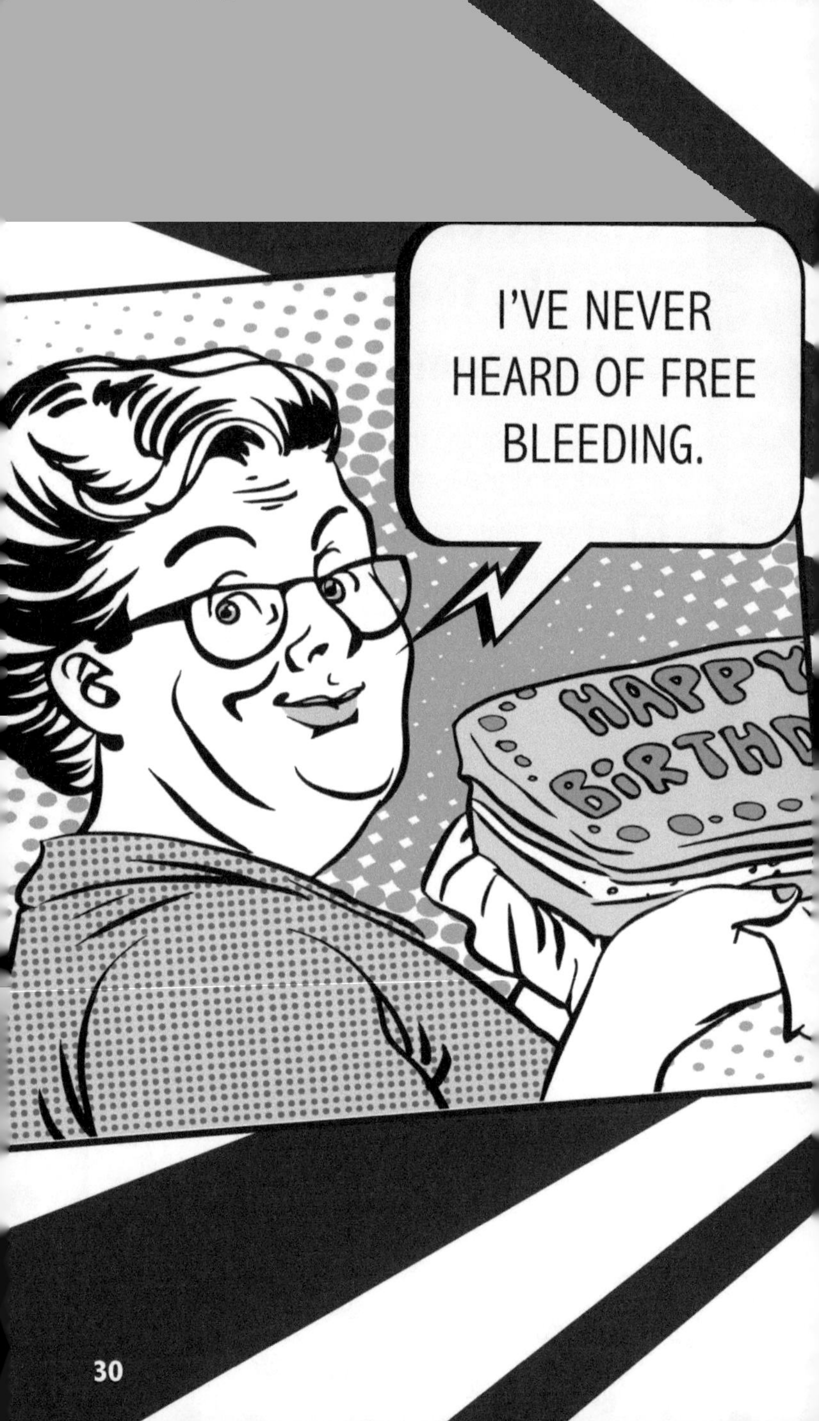

I'VE NEVER HEARD OF FREE BLEEDING.
HAPPY BIRTHD

My lower belly is super sensitive.

But I'm relaxed because I've gotten rid of anything that needed to get out.

IN THE PAST, I would have put in a tampon or used a thick sanitary towel in my pants. Then I would have needed to take a painkiller because I would have pretty bad cramps.

I didn't know my body was getting rid of all the old stuff - and neither my mum nor my grandma or friends had a plan of action to deal with it.

To be able to change this clogged up feeling to one of cosy warmth which spreads through my belly is just amazing.

So I can now experience menstruation as a biological cleanse and even enjoy it. My body makes itself spick and span without any cleaning materials. Amazing!

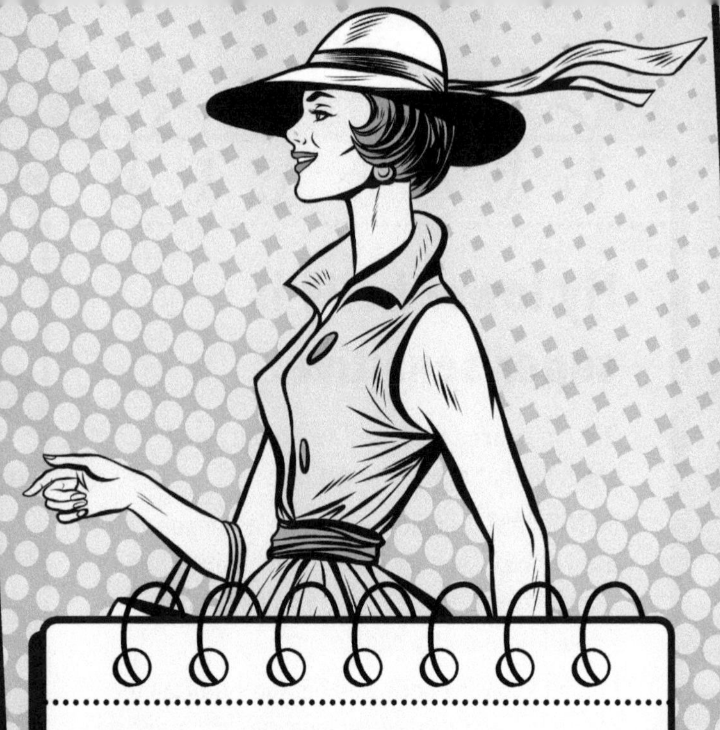

Who needs old mucous membrane?

No one! That's why I'm thinking about how my body is renewing itself internally.

Walking in the fresh air feels good, and the children, as expected, are dawdling, but I don't mind too much today.

I have TIME. Lots of time.

My body enjoys this sense of calm too: It takes care of the cleaning up while I gently support it by going for a nice walk. So everything is coming together well.

What do you like best?

- ☐ The more relaxed I am, the better.
- ☐ I prefer to have lots of peace and time for myself.
- ☐ A bit of movement does me good.
- ☐ I am particularly adventurous and dare to try being product-free on my period in toilets away from home.

- ☐ ....

....

- ☐ ....

....

- ☐ ....

....

Breakfast hunger

10.15AM

When we get home I head straight for the toilet. It feels good, although I could have managed to go for longer.

There is only a teaspoonful of menstrual fluid. The toilet paper in my pants and the sanitary towel underneath are completely clean.

We have a generous breakfast.

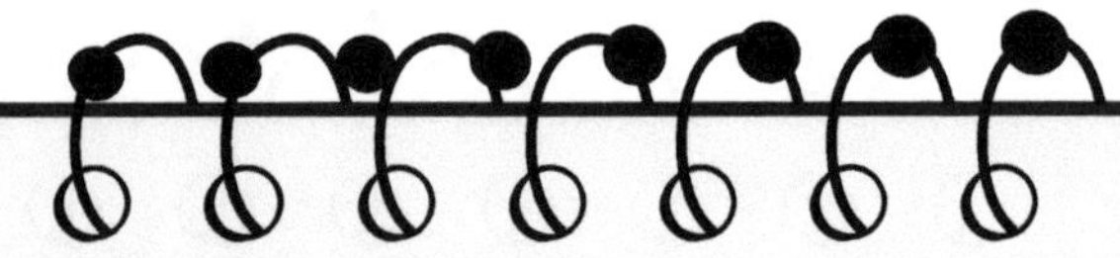

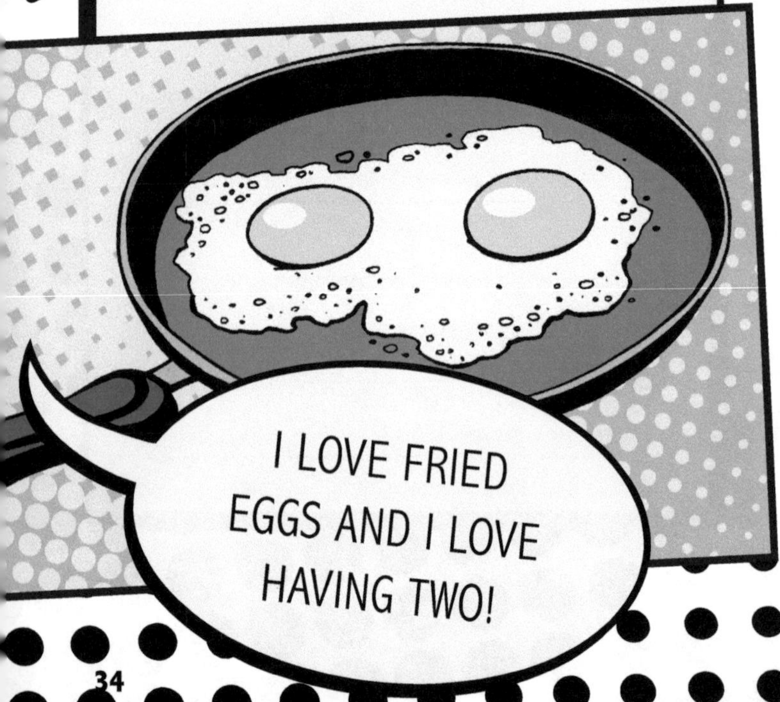

11.15AM

I go to the toilet after breakfast. The toilet paper in my pants is a bit red, but the panty liner underneath has hardly got anything on it.

I release blood by going for a wee, relaxing, and gently rocking forwards and backwards on the toilet. Around two teaspoons of blood come out.

I then go down into a deep squat like I'm going skiing and tilt my pelvis forwards slightly. Some fluid comes out as I change between bearing down and relaxing.

After draining off the viscous fluid, the flow of which has now come to a standstill, I wipe myself off and lay four sheets of folded toilet paper in my pants.

I am completely pain-free and relaxed.

Amazing! Especially as the start of my period used to be particularly plagued by cramps.

Being free feels so good.

11.45AM

I squat down on the carpet in the living room and distractedly flick through a magazine. While my children play peacefully, I realise that I need to do my business again. For the second time today!

I go to the loo and let out what needs to come out. And it's a lot.

The rest of the gassiness thankfully goes away, as this can cause me a fair bit of pain.

11.58AM

Phew. Done. It's been a long time since I've had to sit on the toilet for that long.

After cleaning up, I put the usual four sheets of folded toilet paper into my pants. There's still the panty liner from this morning underneath it.

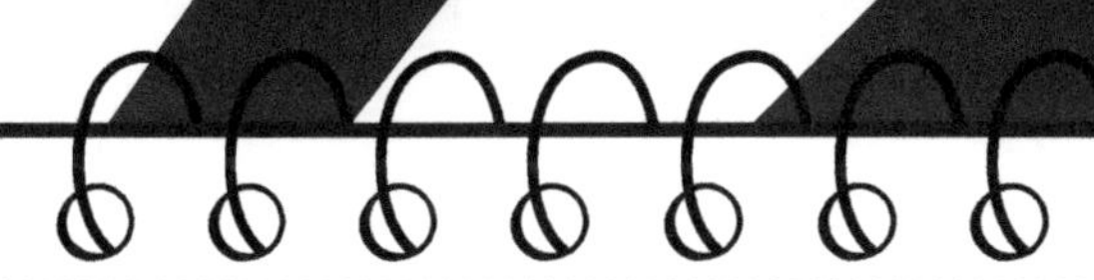

What is the best way to relax?

- ☐ When I have free time and no one wants anything from me.

- ☐ Working.

- ☐ Reading, when I can really get caught up in the story.

- ☐ Watching TV, so I can do something else as well if I want to.

- ☐ ....

  ....

- ☐ ....

  ....

- ☐ ....

  ....

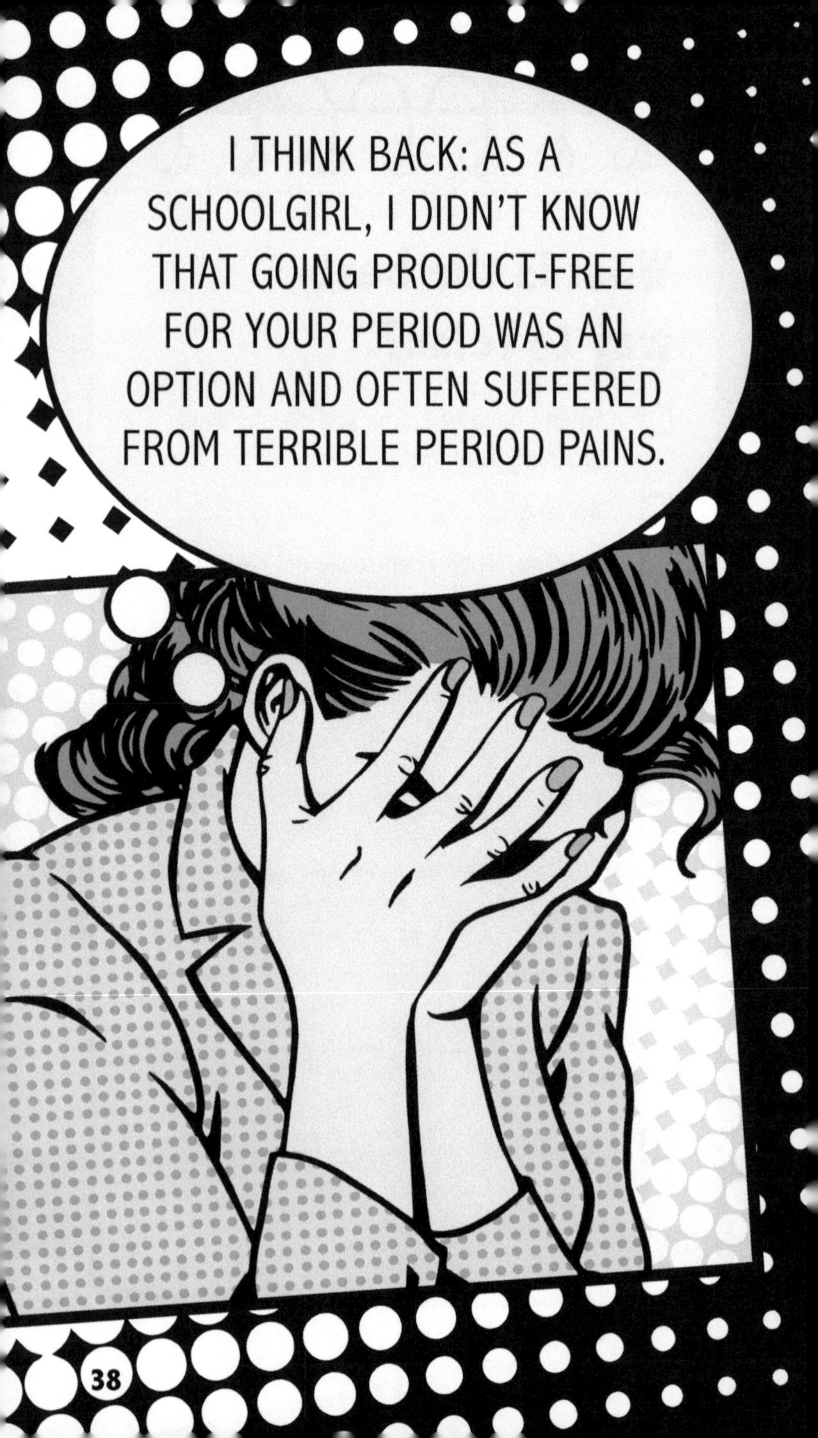

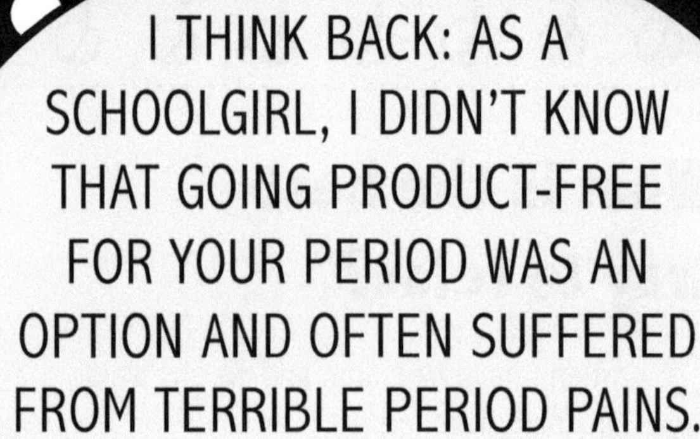

I THINK BACK: AS A SCHOOLGIRL, I DIDN'T KNOW THAT GOING PRODUCT-FREE FOR YOUR PERIOD WAS AN OPTION AND OFTEN SUFFERED FROM TERRIBLE PERIOD PAINS.

How I used to be

I didn't dare go to the school toilets every hour when I was on my period.

What would everyone else think of me?

Aside from that, I didn't yet know about product-free periods and thought you either absorbed all the blood with a sanitary towel or a tampon. There were no menstrual cups at the time, but again, these create an artificial dam where there should really be free passage.

It's important that women know about our periods. After all, it's a prerequisite for having children!

Would men secretly bleed in their trousers or would they make a big show and dance of it and even tell people how much they're bleeding?

It would probably go like this:

"Hey Tom, do you lose 12 litres of blood each month during your period too?" "Only 12? I lose more like 15!"

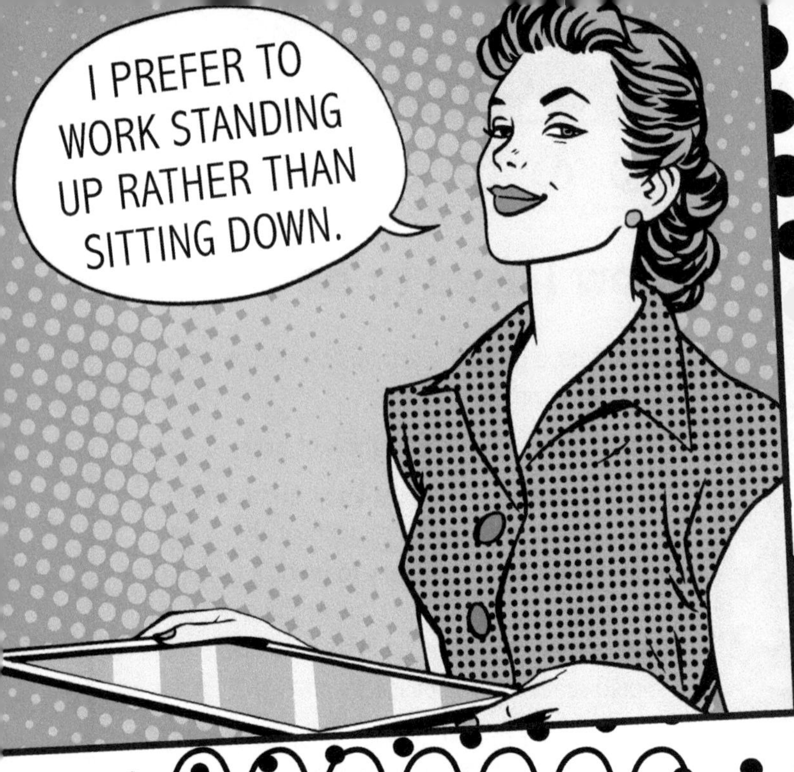

My husband cooked.

1.45PM

I have almost finished everything for my Mars project.

Before lunch I go to the toilet and empty approx. two teaspoons of blood into the loo, the safety toilet paper is almost clean. My stomach has calmed down and it's not as sensitive as it was two hours ago.

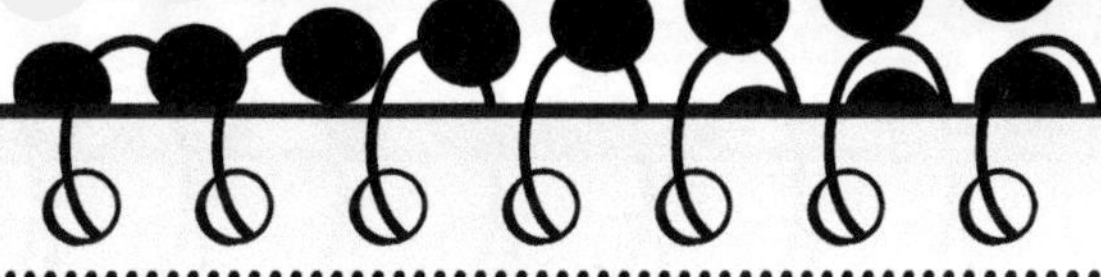

Gone walkabout.

3.20PM

On the toilet, I notice that my toilet paper has moved in my pants and the disposable sanitary towel has got blood on it. What a shame!

I empty out a clump of menstrual discharge and place six folded sheets of TP into my pants.

I'm expecting to use the paper barrier while I'm out and want to protect my pants.

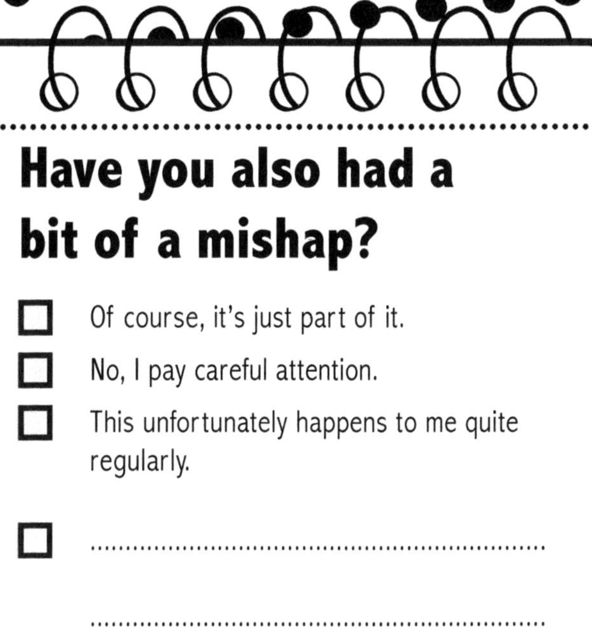

Have you also had a bit of a mishap?

- ☐ Of course, it's just part of it.
- ☐ No, I pay careful attention.
- ☐ This unfortunately happens to me quite regularly.

☐ ....

....

Overflow and stopping leaks
5.05PM

After a long walk it's clear that fluid has built up internally. But I don't feel like I've had a leak yet.

I empty myself out on the toilet. The TP in my pants is barely even red. Draining my menstrual fluid now feels good and takes around 60 seconds. There are several long phases with trickling, dripping, stopping until I reach a real stop.

Yoga and sauna: Tampon management
5.50PM

I'm just cycling to my yoga course which starts at half past six. I empty out again before I go. There's a surprising amount! But 6 sheets of TP as a liner should be enough for the yoga course.

I pack a tampon as I want to go to the sauna afterwards. A few of my friends use a menstrual cup for doing sport during their period, and one uses a sponge. I find normal tampons practical for short-term use.

7.50PM

Yoga is finished. After the twisting, strengthening and deep relaxation, I feel like a new-born.

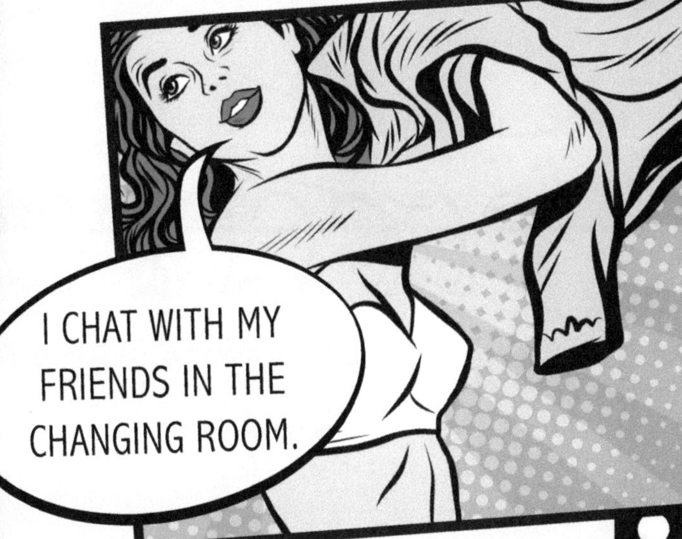

My last visit to the toilet was nearly two hours ago. A lot of blood comes out when I'm in my deep squat, but my toilet paper barrier has almost nothing on it. I'm finished after about a minute and wipe myself off.

I then insert a real tampon because I want to go to the sauna and enjoy it in peace.

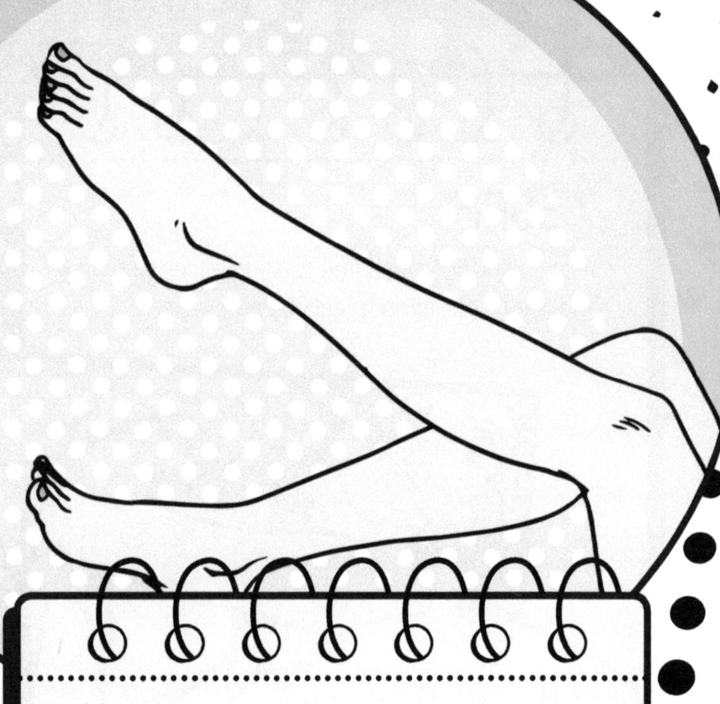

8.30PM

I spent some time in the sauna, sweated a lot and took a long shower. I feel wonderfully refreshed.

I remove the tampon in the toilet. It is half soaked with blood. I quickly dispose of it in the small bin which is attached to the toilet wall for this purpose. Thankfully, I don't have to look in there often, it's pretty disgusting...

I lay four sheets of folded toilet paper into my pants. That's enough to last until I'm home.

Now to quickly blow-dry my hair. Done. I cycle home.

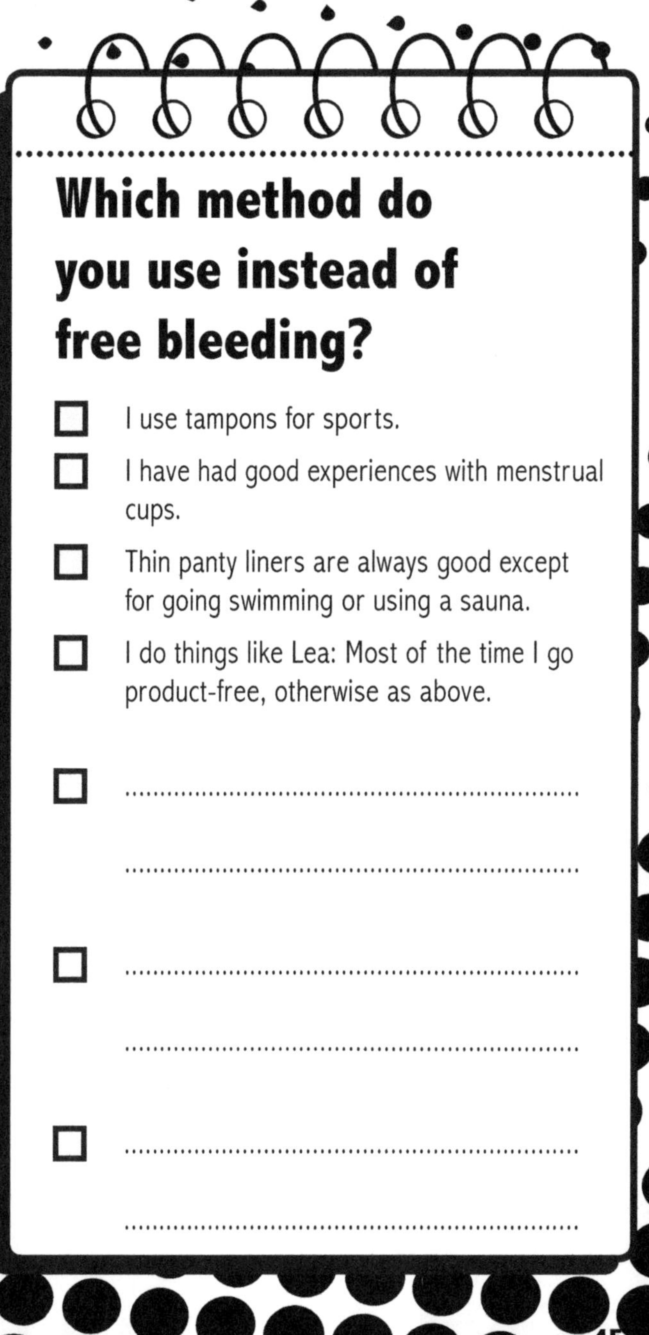

Which method do you use instead of free bleeding?

- ☐ I use tampons for sports.
- ☐ I have had good experiences with menstrual cups.
- ☐ Thin panty liners are always good except for going swimming or using a sauna.
- ☐ I do things like Lea: Most of the time I go product-free, otherwise as above.
- ☐ ....
- ☐ ....
- ☐ ....

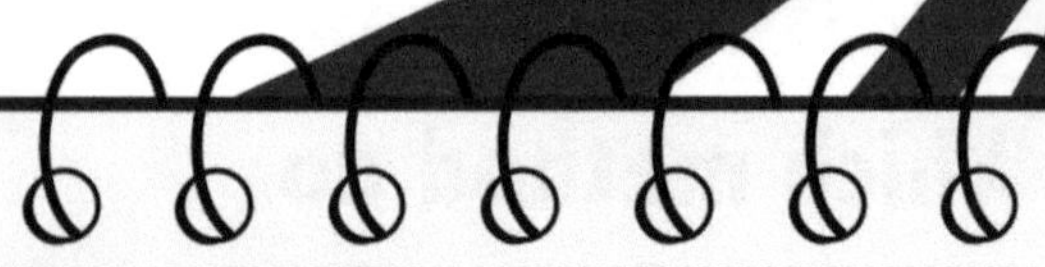

Back home
9PM

I write in my period diary. I then really need to wee, the aftermath of using the sauna. Some menstrual blood comes out too.

Now just a little bite to eat and then it's a well-deserved rest watching TV on the sofa with my husband. Periods can be nice and relaxed when everything runs in a controlled way.

Getting ready to sleep
10.50PM

Brushing my teeth on tip-toes and going to the loo again before going to sleep. Very little blood comes out.

I place eight folded sheets of TP into my pants. I know that I'll feel "heavy" during the night, but I quickly head to the toilet after waking up. Thankfully it's just a few steps away from the bed.

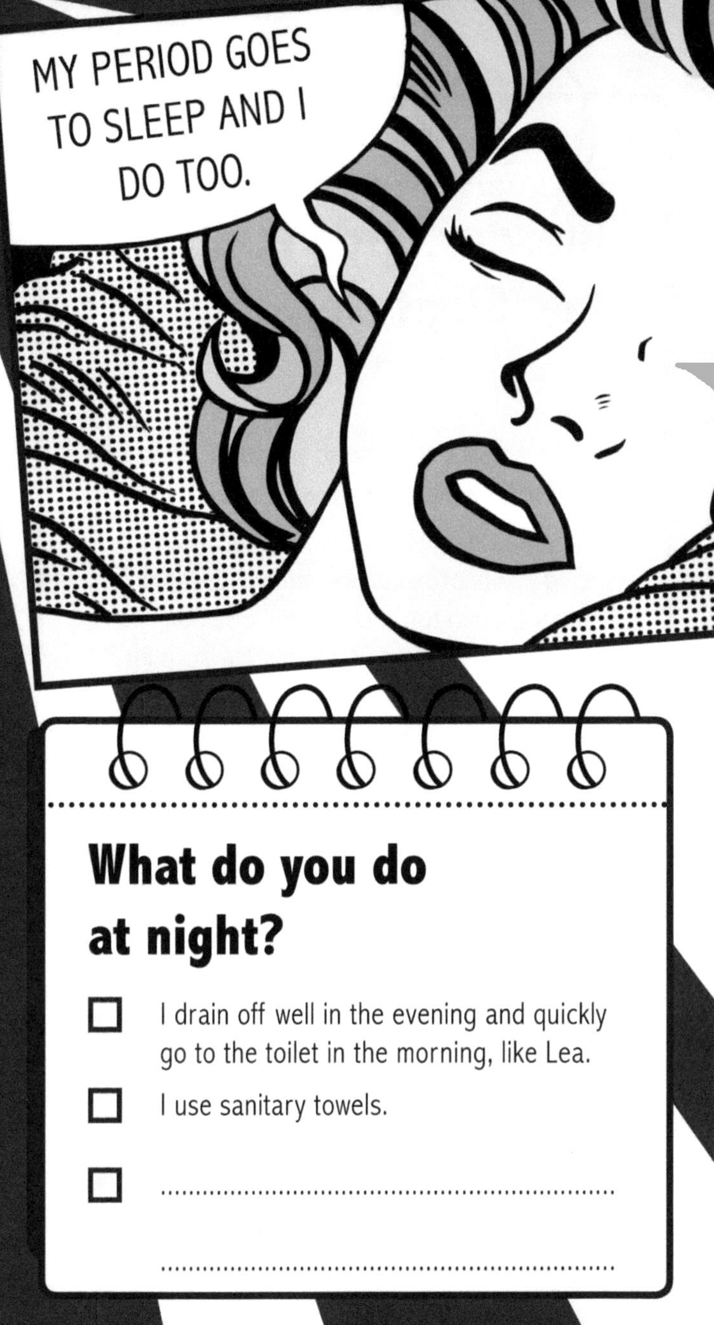

What do you do at night?

- ☐ I drain off well in the evening and quickly go to the toilet in the morning, like Lea.
- ☐ I use sanitary towels.
- ☐ ....

Tuesday, 3rd cycle day: Slept well

7.35AM

There's no school today, so we can sleep longer. Even the little night owl stays in bed.

As I go to the toilet, I am looking forward to seeing plenty of blood and am not disappointed. There's around two tablespoons of blood which quickly flow out of me in a few seconds. I accelerate the emptying process by bearing down, relaxing, bearing down and relaxing.

I clean myself up and place four sheets of folded toilet paper in my pants.

8.05AM

I go to the toilet again when brushing my teeth. Only a little bit comes out. Four sheets of TP in my knickers.

It's walkies with the dogs after breakfast.

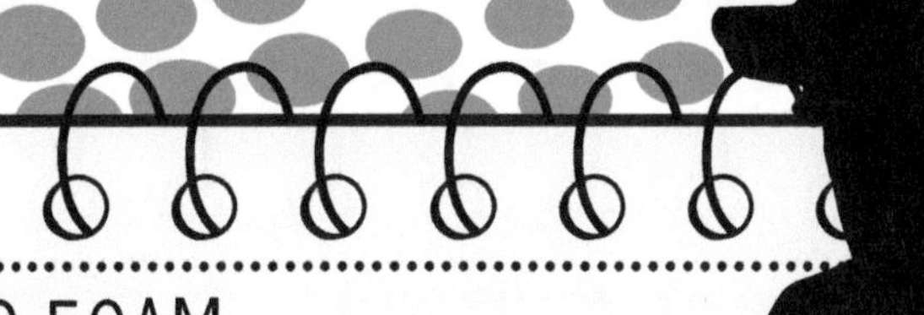

9.50AM

A large amount of menstrual discharge comes out at home. I see that there's some blood on the toilet paper. I put four sheets of TP in my knickers.

To the train station
11.30AM

The toilet paper is nearly clean. I empty out, even though hardly anything comes out, as a precaution because I have to go to the train station. For security, I put a panty liner under the six folded sheets of TP.

And on the go?

☐ I use sanitary towels, better safe than sorry.

☐ I prefer to use tampons.

☐ I find a place to empty out.

☐ ....

....

Off to the stables

2.30PM

Three hours later, I'm back home. It is half past two by the time I go to the toilet. I want to empty out again before going to the riding stables.

A large amount of menstrual discharge comes out without dripping. The toilet paper has hardly any blood on it and the panty liner is clear. I put just four sheets of TP in my knickers as there's a nice toilet at the stables, if I need to use it.

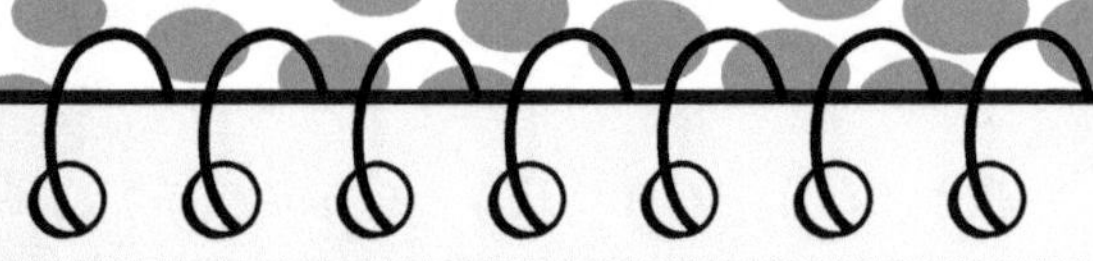

5.30PM

We're back from the stables. One to two smaller blobs of menstrual discharge come out in the toilet at home.

The toilet paper is white, as is the panty liner. I use just three folded sheets of TP and use the inserted paper to wipe off.

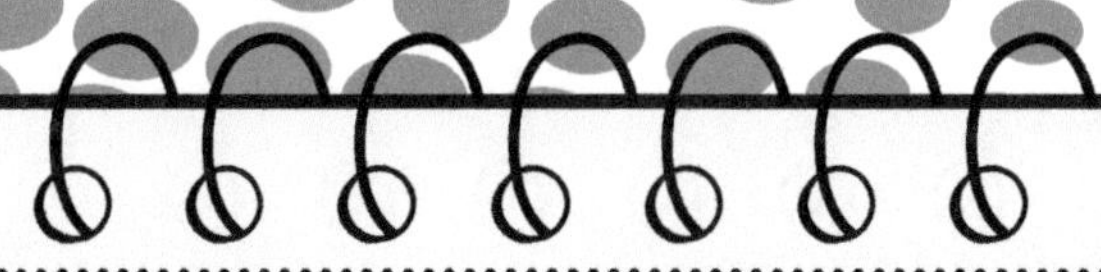

7.10PM

There's more yoga luxury ahead. I wipe myself off as there's nothing coming out and put two sheets of TP in my knickers.

Self-rolled tampon

9PM

I only have a little to empty out after yoga. I grab a sheet of toilet paper, fold it in half and twist it into my own "auxiliary tampon" for the sauna. I leave a bit of it sticking out so that I can easily remove it afterwards.

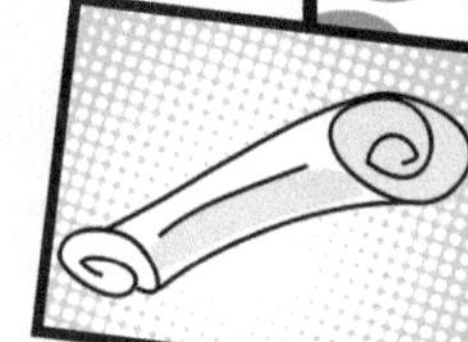

9.15PM

I remove the auxiliary tampon after using the sauna. It is only half soaked in blood. I then have an ice cold shower, go to the toilet and put two sheets of TP in my knickers. I get dressed and go home.

10.30PM

As always, I go to the toilet before going to sleep. I have nothing else to drain off and put four sheets of TP in my knickers.

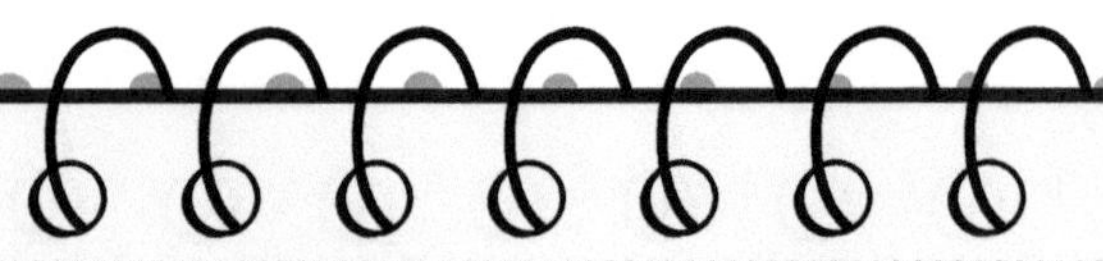

Wednesday, 4th cycle day: Spotting starts

6.30AM

School's back on again ... get up, yawn!

On the toilet I see that the toilet paper has remained clean overnight. It's only just the fourth day of my cycle – was that really everything?

I wrap my forefinger in toilet paper and carefully insert it: The menstrual blood is somewhat more watery and there is nothing to actively empty out.

I still put three folded sheets of TP into my pants as a precaution, as I assume there will be spotting.

8.40AM

There's a red-brown smear on the TP. It's not possible to empty anything out. I replace the TP with two sheets as I'm staying at home.

11.30AM

More smears. I replace the virtually clean TP with three sheets as I have a bit of a trip to get to the nursery.

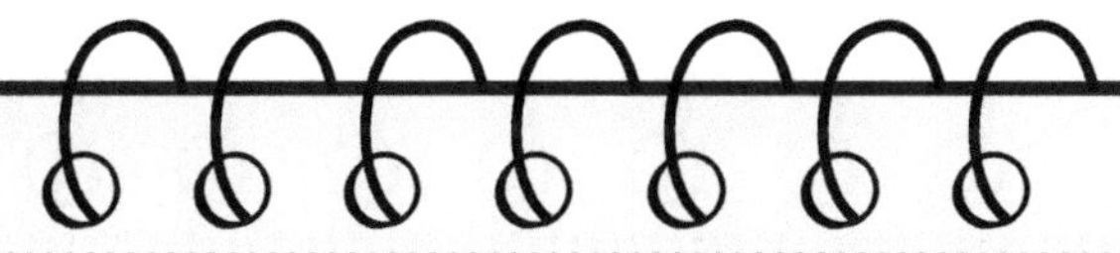

Bike trip to the countryside

3.30PM

The weather is nice and we cycle to the river. We have picnic things in our bags.

I go to the toilet before we leave. When bearing down a small lump of menstrual discharge comes out. After all, it was four hours ago since I was last on the loo.

As I don't expect much more to come out, I think three sheets of folded TP is enough. There will always be a bush along the way if there's an emergency.

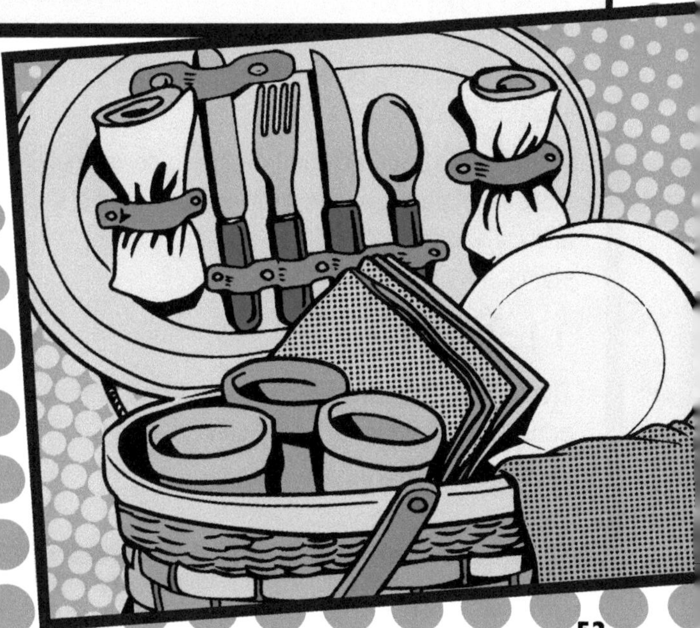

6.45PM

The trip was lovely and I only needed to take one stop on the way to empty out.

The TP in my pants is red-brown but dry. No real draining is possible due to the slight spotting. I place three folded sheets of TP into my pants to protect my underwear.

My husband is at home. I go off to the furniture store as I need a lamp.

It's coming to an end.

8.30PM

I'm back home. As before, I have some light spotting which doesn't drip.

The TP has stayed dry. So I decide to do without more toilet paper, as I'm wearing black knickers anyway and am not really all that fussy about stains.

11.30PM

The spotting is lessening, my pants are dry. My period has come to an end. I don't need any TP for the night time.

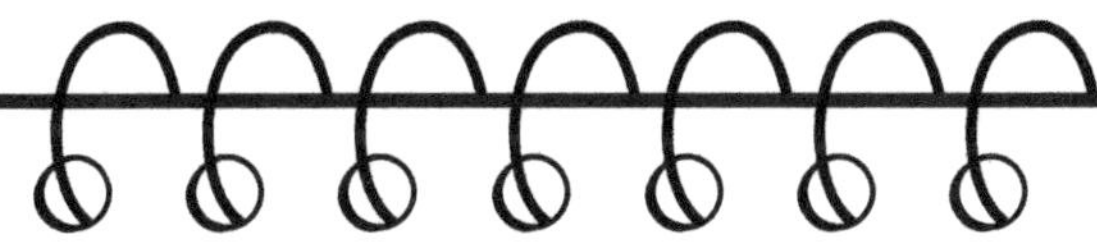

My period is almost over ...

- ☐ I find that I still have a bit of spotting for a couple of days afterwards.

- ☐ I bleed fairly heavily nearly all the way to the end of the period.

- ☐ Like Lea, I find that I can almost do without TP inserts at the end.

- ☐ I don't care about the last couple of days of my period if I'm wearing black pants.

- ☐ ....

  ....

- ☐ ....

  ....

- ☐ ....

  ....

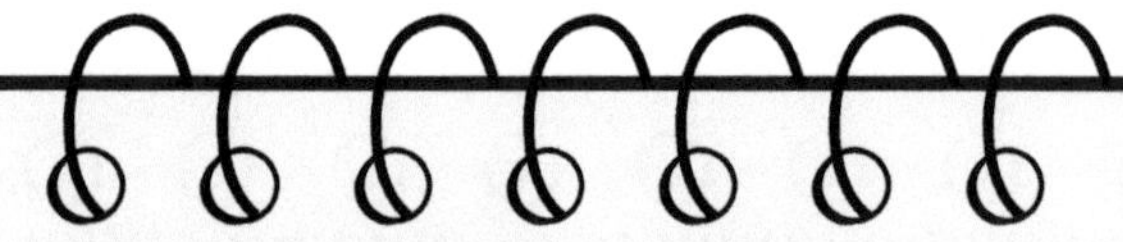

Thursday, 5th cycle day: Almost finished

6.30AM

My pants have remained dry, even without a TP insert.

However, when I go to the loo in the morning I still notice fairly heavy spotting which I wipe off. There's nothing to empty out. I do without a TP insert.

8AM

The spotting is lessening, the blood is lighter. I wipe myself off thoroughly and still do without a TP insert.
I'm off to the nursery and to go shopping.

One last little bit

10AM

Great! Once home I managed to get out a little lump of menstrual discharge! :-)
The spotting is very light and I don't need a TP insert.

Finally had a bowel movement again

11.55AM

Just before twelve I finally had a bowel movement again.

I remember that after giving birth it also took a few days for my bowels to start working again.

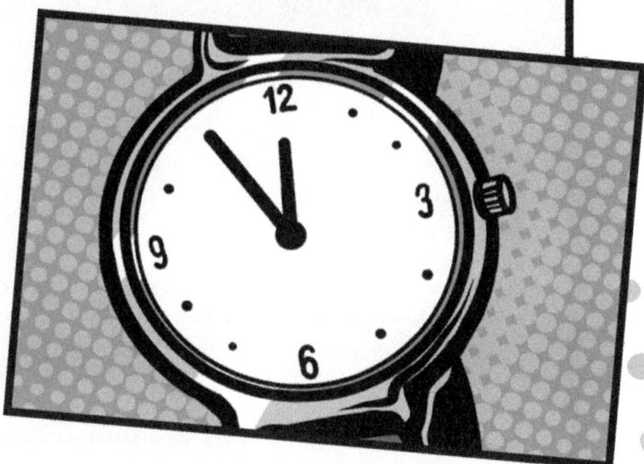

1.50PM, 3.30PM, 5.10PM

I didn't actually have to go to the toilet this often. There is less and less bleeding, there is only some dripping red mucus in the evening when I try to empty out.

The clean up is almost over.

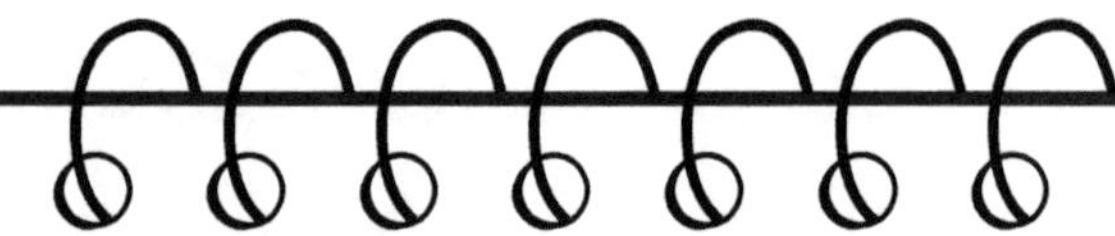

What have you learned about your digestion?

- ☐ Nothing much, I already knew it pretty well beforehand.

- ☐ Digestion and my period go hand in hand. That's interesting!

- ☐ I digest a lot at the beginning of my period and then there's a break.

- ☐ Being gassy during my period is particularly painful.

- ☐ ....

  ....

- ☐ ....

  ....

- ☐ ....

  ....

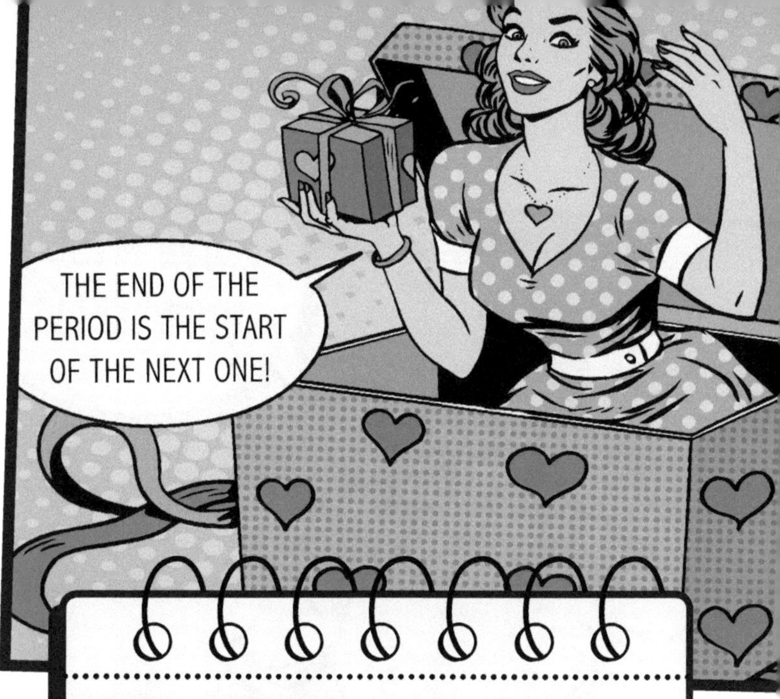

6th and 7th cycle days: An end and a new beginning

FRIDAY

There is still some rusty brown mucus during the day. I'm not bothered by it.

SATURDAY

There is some light reddish mucus in the morning. By noon this has also gone, even after probing.

Free bleeding is over and a new time of fertility and development begins.

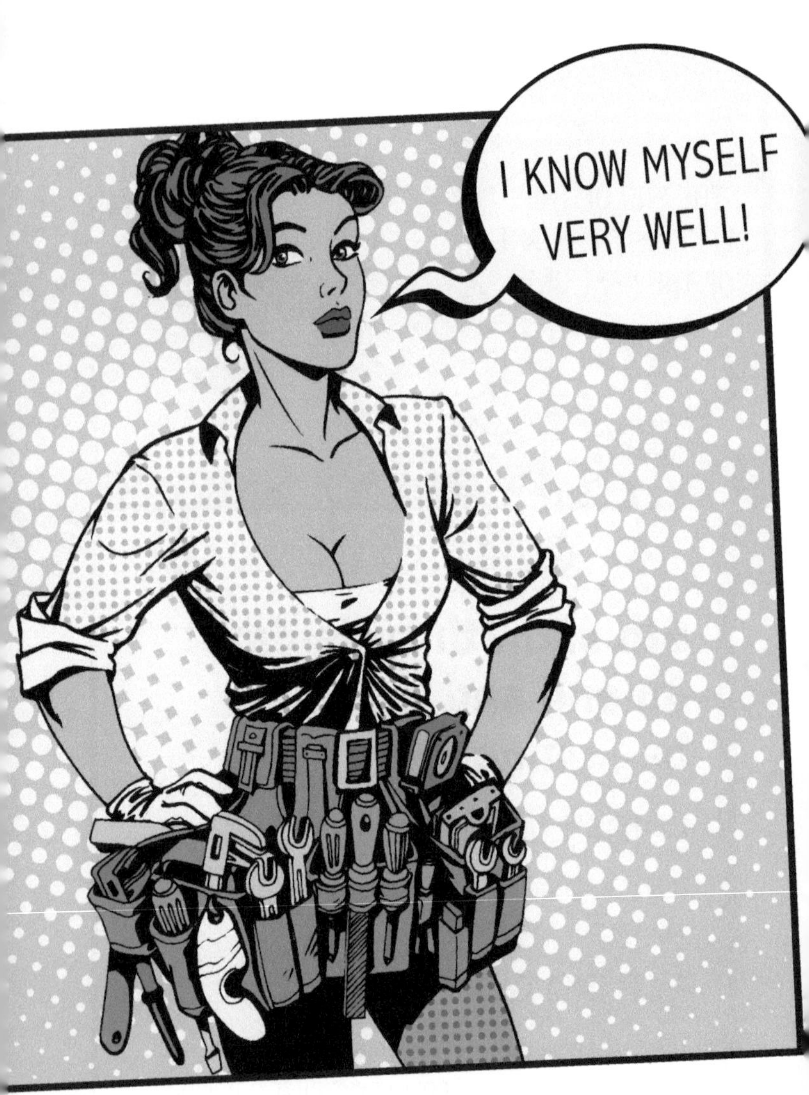
I KNOW MYSELF
VERY WELL!

Your free bleeding and its phases

Now create your own period log to learn about a product-free period and practice it in peace. Familiarise yourself with the various MENSTRUAL PHASES to understand what strength of flow to expect.

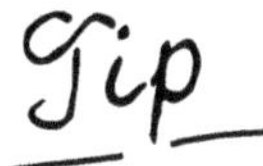

*   If you regularly take your morning WAKING TEMPERATURE, the drop in temperature will tell you when to expect the start of your period.

*   COMBINED with monitoring your vaginal mucus, you can also prevent or plan pregnancy if you follow the rules very carefully. This method is called the "Sympto-thermal method" because you are looking for symptoms and measuring your temperature. Another term for this is "NFP" — Natural Family Planning. Get a special exercise book if you are interested in this method.

Whatever you plan to do: Being an expert on your period is just as good an idea for young girls as it is for older women who want to prevent or encourage pregnancy. As a woman, you should always know what's going on in your body.

Period phase 0: The feeling that something is going to happen

PMS, pre-menstrual syndrome. It sounds dangerous, and it can be – mostly to those around you ;-)

Have you already heard of it? For example, when someone around you talked about "having PMS" in the days before their period and was talking about a certain female and how irritable they were?

It's not surprising you're irritable. There's a major hormonal change coming because all of the construction work and fertility your body fostered has been for nothing. All that courting has done nothing: The egg will now be expelled, along with its constructed mobile home in your uterus, by which we mean the lovely, fertile mucus membrane.

Period phase 1: Shedding begins

Bleeding usually starts slowly with fresh blood which you will notice on your toilet paper.

In this phase:

*   Gassiness which can even be felt the day before the shedding.

A (large) bowel movement often takes place at this time. Just like before giving birth, the body is thoroughly cleaning itself and making the paths as clear as possible.

Period phase 2: The floodgates are opened

Now it's on to the preserved tissue, because all of the used tissue has to be removed.

In this phase:

*   The lower abdomen is very sensitive.

*   The force of the emptying out is reminiscent of a real birth, there's no holding back anymore.

This phase usually takes place on the 1st and 2nd days of your period.

You might now feel just as sensitive as your lower belly and blockages (tampons and the like) can particularly hinder being able to excrete without experiencing pain.

If you notice that you tend to have stomach cramps, then try sitting relaxed on the toilet and letting everything down below flow out.

Including gas, because this is often unpleasant and can cause very severe pains.

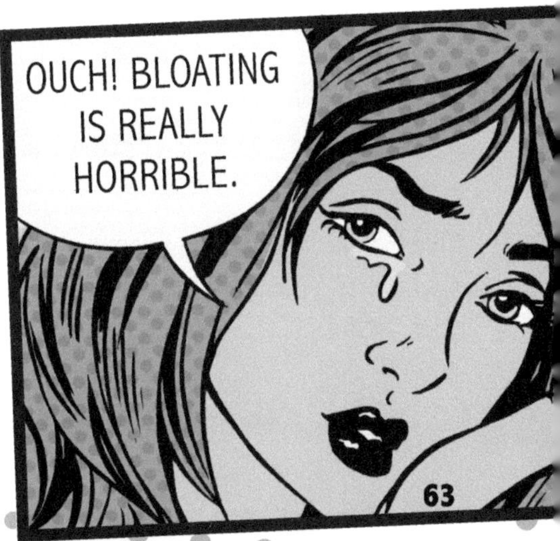

Period phase 3: Orderly clean up

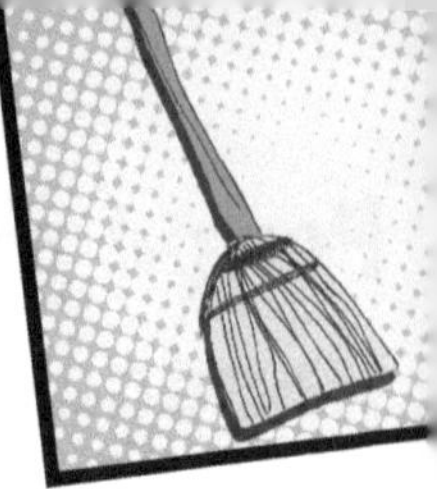

Following the quick "birthing phase" comes the carefully conducted "cleaning phase", just like the post-birth vaginal discharge after giving birth.

In this phase:

*   The cleaning is thorough and comprehensive.

*   All parts still in the uterus are removed and anything no longer useful is disposed of.

The cleaning phase usually takes place on the 3rd and 4th days of your period.

Period phase 4: Leaking and spotting

The final credits roll once the uterus has been thoroughly emptied out and cleaned.

In this phase:

*   Just like a film at the cinema, the credits can last for some time.

*   There is still some dripping and spotting during the final stage.

This menstrual phase can sometimes overlap with period phase 3 and usually takes place on the 5th and 6th day of your period.

Period phase 5: Clean mucus lining is restored

The spotting merges with the clean mucus to form the new basis for a fertile period.

The following applies: After one period is before the next period, because if the clean and later on fertile mucus membrane is not used for pregnancy, the unfertilised egg automatically leads to new shedding bleeding.

Good to know:

* The already mentioned "Sympto-thermal method" (i.e. the combination of mucus monitoring and temperature measurement) starts from 6 infertile days after the beginning of the cycle. Then, if you have unprotected sex, the race to fertilise the egg starts again.

* So you should be careful and know that you can become pregnant relatively early in your cycle! Sperm can survive in the fertile mucus for several days and you never know when you will ovulate next.

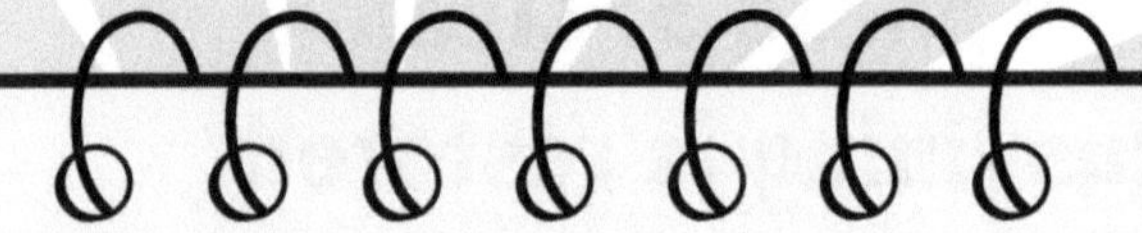

Now record your free bleeding!

Find out which period days and phases apply to you and how you can best implement the product-free period in your life.

It's helpful to note down the times of your observations and you can then quickly see how long the individual phases last.

A mental schedule helps to protect you from unpleasant surprises.

So, if you're practicing free bleeding, you know in advance how often you will need to visit the toilet in order to stay dry.

Or, if you are planning to use hygiene products economically and in a targeted way, e.g. if you want to go swimming, have a test or will not have access to a toilet for several hours at work.

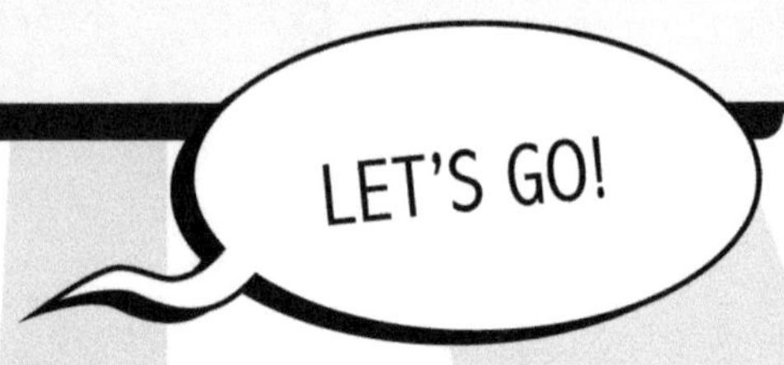

DAY: .... **/** .... 20......

CYCLE DAY: .... PERIOD PHASE: ....

HYGIENE PRODUCT(S): ....

.... : .... Time

☐ Empty out ☐ Menstrual discharge ☐ Spotting

.... : .... Time

☐ Empty out ☐ Menstrual discharge ☐ Spotting

.... : .... Time

☐ Empty out ☐ Menstrual discharge ☐ Spotting

.... : .... Time

☐ Empty out ☐ Menstrual discharge ☐ Spotting

DAY: .... **/** .... 20......

CYCLE DAY: .... PERIOD PHASE: ....

HYGIENE PRODUCT(S): ....

.... : .... Time

☐ Empty out ☐ Menstrual discharge ☐ Spotting

.... : .... Time

☐ Empty out ☐ Menstrual discharge ☐ Spotting

.... : .... Time

☐ Empty out ☐ Menstrual discharge ☐ Spotting

.... : .... Time

☐ Empty out ☐ Menstrual discharge ☐ Spotting

DAY: .... / .... 20......

CYCLE DAY: .... PERIOD PHASE: ....

HYGIENE PRODUCT(S): ....

.... : .... Time

☐ Empty out ☐ Menstrual discharge ☐ Spotting

.... : .... Time

☐ Empty out ☐ Menstrual discharge ☐ Spotting

.... : .... Time

☐ Empty out ☐ Menstrual discharge ☐ Spotting

.... : .... Time

☐ Empty out ☐ Menstrual discharge ☐ Spotting

DAY: .... **/** .... 20......

CYCLE DAY: .... PERIOD PHASE: ....

HYGIENE PRODUCT(S): ....

.... : .... Time

☐ Empty out ☐ Menstrual discharge ☐ Spotting

.... : .... Time

☐ Empty out ☐ Menstrual discharge ☐ Spotting

.... : .... Time

☐ Empty out ☐ Menstrual discharge ☐ Spotting

.... : .... Time

☐ Empty out ☐ Menstrual discharge ☐ Spotting

DAY: .... **/** ..... **.** ...... 20......

CYCLE DAY: .... PERIOD PHASE: ....

HYGIENE PRODUCT(S): ....

.... : .... Time

☐ Empty out ☐ Menstrual discharge ☐ Spotting

....

.... : .... Time

☐ Empty out ☐ Menstrual discharge ☐ Spotting

....

.... : .... Time

☐ Empty out ☐ Menstrual discharge ☐ Spotting

....

.... : .... Time

☐ Empty out ☐ Menstrual discharge ☐ Spotting

....

DAY: .... / .... 20......

CYCLE DAY: .... PERIOD PHASE: ....

HYGIENE PRODUCT(S): ....

.... : .... Time

☐ Empty out ☐ Menstrual discharge ☐ Spotting

.... : .... Time

☐ Empty out ☐ Menstrual discharge ☐ Spotting

.... : .... Time

☐ Empty out ☐ Menstrual discharge ☐ Spotting

.... : .... Time

☐ Empty out ☐ Menstrual discharge ☐ Spotting

DAY: .... **/** .... 20......

CYCLE DAY: .... PERIOD PHASE: ....

HYGIENE PRODUCT(S): ....

.... : .... Time

☐ Empty out ☐ Menstrual discharge ☐ Spotting

.... : .... Time

☐ Empty out ☐ Menstrual discharge ☐ Spotting

.... : .... Time

☐ Empty out ☐ Menstrual discharge ☐ Spotting

.... : .... Time

☐ Empty out ☐ Menstrual discharge ☐ Spotting

DAY: .... **/** .... .20......

CYCLE DAY: .... PERIOD PHASE: ....

HYGIENE PRODUCT(S): ....

.... : .... Time

☐ Empty out ☐ Menstrual discharge ☐ Spotting

....

.... : .... Time

☐ Empty out ☐ Menstrual discharge ☐ Spotting

....

.... : .... Time

☐ Empty out ☐ Menstrual discharge ☐ Spotting

....

.... : .... Time

☐ Empty out ☐ Menstrual discharge ☐ Spotting

....

DAY: .... **/** .... .20......

CYCLE DAY: .... PERIOD PHASE: ....

HYGIENE PRODUCT(S): ....

.... : .... Time

☐ Empty out ☐ Menstrual discharge ☐ Spotting

.... : .... Time

☐ Empty out ☐ Menstrual discharge ☐ Spotting

.... : .... Time

☐ Empty out ☐ Menstrual discharge ☐ Spotting

.... : .... Time

☐ Empty out ☐ Menstrual discharge ☐ Spotting

DAY: ..../ .... 20......

CYCLE DAY: .... PERIOD PHASE: ....

HYGIENE PRODUCT(S): ....

.... : .... Time

☐ Empty out ☐ Menstrual discharge ☐ Spotting

.... : .... Time

☐ Empty out ☐ Menstrual discharge ☐ Spotting

.... : .... Time

☐ Empty out ☐ Menstrual discharge ☐ Spotting

.... : .... Time

☐ Empty out ☐ Menstrual discharge ☐ Spotting

DAY: .... **/** ..... **.** ...... 20......

CYCLE DAY: .... PERIOD PHASE: ....

HYGIENE PRODUCT(S): ....

.... : .... Time

☐ Empty out ☐ Menstrual discharge ☐ Spotting

.... : .... Time

☐ Empty out ☐ Menstrual discharge ☐ Spotting

.... : .... Time

☐ Empty out ☐ Menstrual discharge ☐ Spotting

.... : .... Time

☐ Empty out ☐ Menstrual discharge ☐ Spotting

DAY: .... **/** .... .20......

CYCLE DAY: .... PERIOD PHASE: ....

HYGIENE PRODUCT(S): ....

.... : .... Time

☐ Empty out ☐ Menstrual discharge ☐ Spotting

.... : .... Time

☐ Empty out ☐ Menstrual discharge ☐ Spotting

.... : .... Time

☐ Empty out ☐ Menstrual discharge ☐ Spotting

.... : .... Time

☐ Empty out ☐ Menstrual discharge ☐ Spotting

DAY: .... **/** ......·......·20......

CYCLE DAY: .... PERIOD PHASE: ....

HYGIENE PRODUCT(S): ....

.... : .... Time

☐ Empty out ☐ Menstrual discharge ☐ Spotting

.... : .... Time

☐ Empty out ☐ Menstrual discharge ☐ Spotting

.... : .... Time

☐ Empty out ☐ Menstrual discharge ☐ Spotting

.... : .... Time

☐ Empty out ☐ Menstrual discharge ☐ Spotting

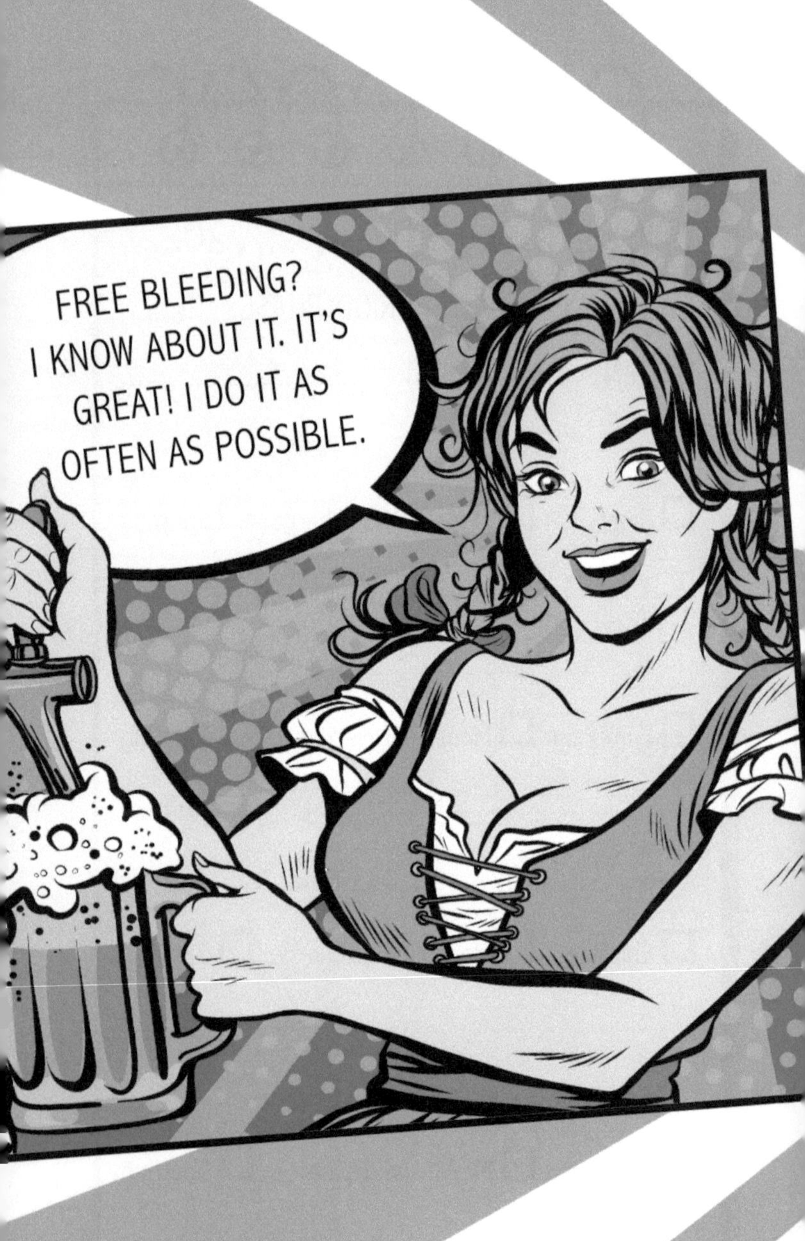

FREE BLEEDING? I KNOW ABOUT IT. IT'S GREAT! I DO IT AS OFTEN AS POSSIBLE.

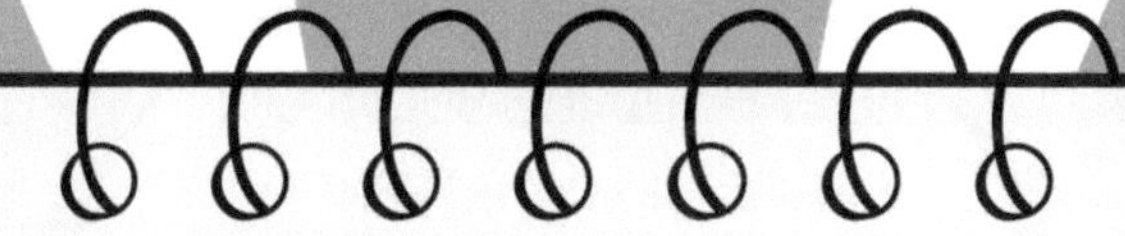

Committing to free bleeding without products?

Just tell your friends, acquaintances and colleagues about your new method — the PRODUCT-FREE PERIOD. Encourage other women to take the time to menstruate freely during their period.

You're sure to have some ideas on how to tell people about free bleeding.

☐ "I menstruate freely and need a toilet now."

☐ "Is anyone else on their period?"

☐ ....

....

☐ ....

....

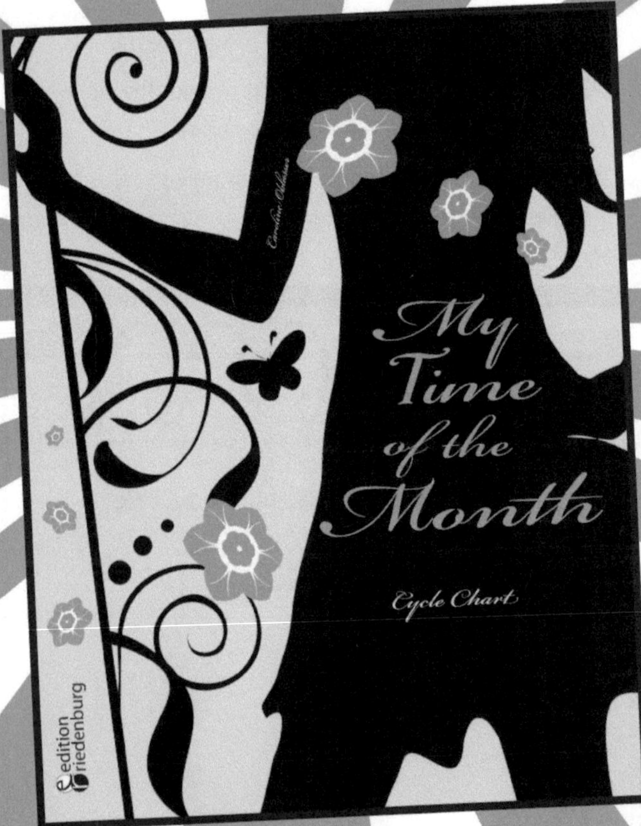

LEA'S FAVOURITE BOOKS CAN
BE FOUND IN (INTERNET)
BOOKSHOPS AND AT
EDITIONRIEDENBURG.AT

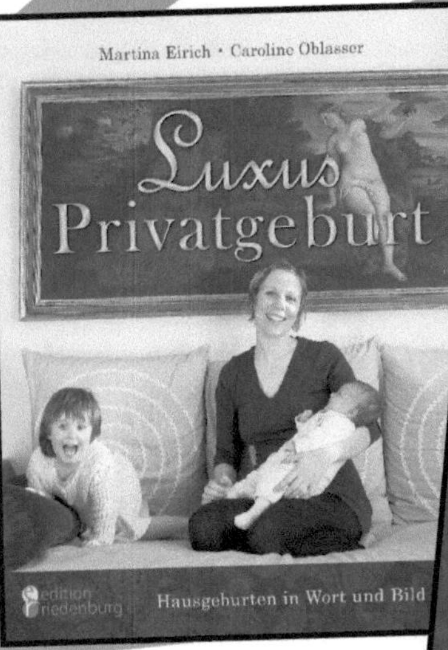

LUXURY PRIVATE BIRTH

HOME BIRTH IN WORDS AND IMAGES

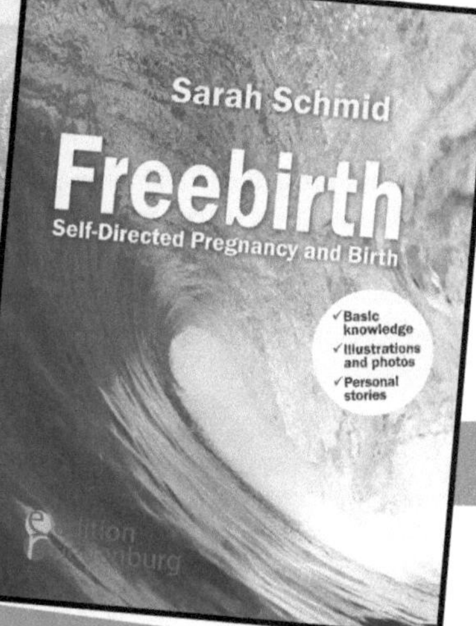

FREEBIRTH

SELF-DIRECTED PREGNANCY AND BIRTH

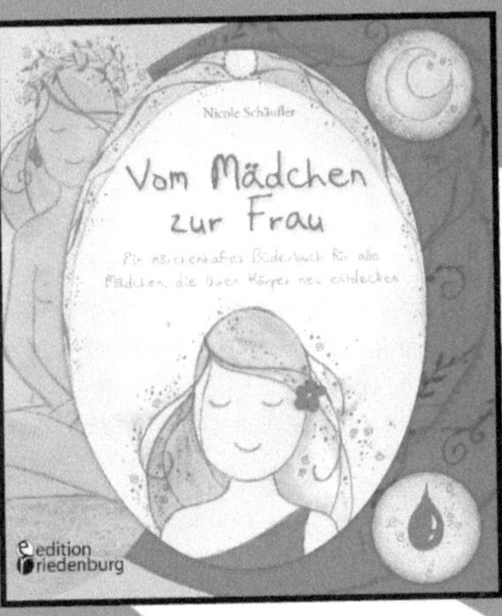

FROM GIRL TO WOMAN

A FAIRY TALE PICTURE BOOK FOR ALL GIRLS WHO WANT TO DISCOVER THEIR BODIES

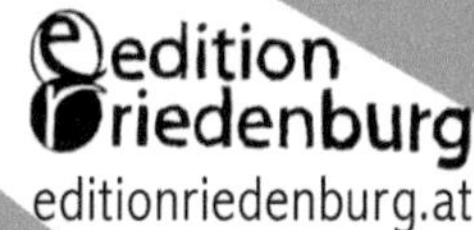

Bibliographic information at the Deutsche Nationalbibliothek: The Deutsche Nationalbibliothek records this publication in the Deutschen Nationalbibliographie; detailed bibliographic information can be obtained online at: http://dnb.d-nb.de.

1st Edition   November 2016
© 2016   edition riedenburg

Published originally under the title "Die freie Mens — Leas COMIC-TAGEBUCH für eine schmerzfreie Regel ohne Binden, Tampons und Co" (© edition riedenburg 2016)

Publisher's information
edition riedenburg, Anton-Hochmuth-Strasse 8, 5020 Salzburg, Austria

Internet   www.editionriedenburg.at
E-Mail   verlag@editionriedenburg.at
Editors   Dr. Heike Wolter, Regensburg; Carla Oblasser, Salzburg
Translation   tolingo.com
Illustrations   The following illustrations come from Fotolia.com:
© studiostoks: Cover woman, waitress, space babe, woman with gas in the past, woman with tool belt, woman in the box, watch, picnic basket, woman working standing with tablet in hand, sobbing woman, fried eggs, woman with hat, grandma with birthday cake, woman near washing machine, kissing couple, woman with diary, two women having a conversation, woman in the ball gown, woman with protective helmet, toilet, individual speech bubbles, large lips with speech bubble
© Alexander Pokusay: Horse, sleeping woman, dog, hand with toilet paper
© rogistok: Naked legs
© reineg: Illustration of the menstrual cycle

Composition and layout by edition riedenburg

ISBN 978-3-903085-64-0

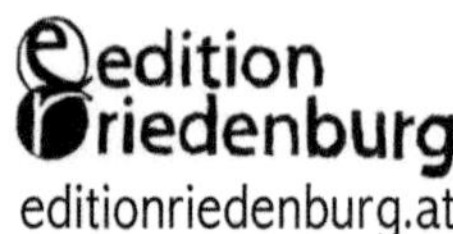